The physical examination

To Diane and Irene,
Paul and Frank

The physical examination

An atlas for general practice

**L. Lodewick
and A.D.G. Gunn**

with a Foreword by
Prof. Robert Greenblatt
Medical College of Georgia

Published, in association with
Hastings Hilton Publishers Limited,
by

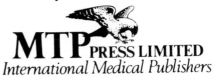

Published, in association with
Hastings Hilton Publishers Limited
London, by

MTP Press Limited
Falcon House
Lancaster, England

ISBN 0–85200–395–1

Printed in the USA

Foreword

What a refreshing experience it is for one who has practiced medicine for quite a few decades to be reminded again of the basics in the physical examination of a patient – to look, to touch, and to listen. Drs. Lodewick and Gunn, with simple illustrations and an economy of words, present the medical student and the student of medicine, i.e. the clinician, digestible tit-bits of the very essence of physical diagnosis. The book is a mine of information – equipping the fledgling physician with necessary know-how and reacquainting the general practitioner of methods with which he once was cognizant or bringing new and useful technics to his attention. I was particularly fascinated by the simple step by step instructions that enable any physician to do a neurological examination and learn how readily CNS disturbances manifest themselves in visible ways, i.e. 'failure of adduction of the thumb is absent in patients with lesions of the pyramidal tract if the middle finger is passively flipped as far as possible at the metacarpophalangeal joint' (page 46, illustration #6). The book abounds with brief informative tips. In palpation of the common carotid artery 'do not palpate the arteries on both sides at the same time; carotid pressure can cause a loss of consciousness (and even cardiac arrest); when trying to differentiate thyroid enlargements from other growths remember that aberrant thyroid gland tissue moves together with swallowing movements'.

Because the mortality rate from mammary cancer has not improved in 40 years, the onus now rests on the primary physician to make the diagnosis early. This goal can be reached by utilizing such modalities as mammography, thermography, and sonography but above all by a meticulous examination. Particularly praiseworthy is the section to help detect palpable anomalies in the breast and the regional lymph nodes.

Medical healing is an art; physiologic interpretation of disease a science, but the procedure necessary for a meaningful physical examination is a skill. Every student and general practitioner can readily improve his technics and acquire proficiency in this aspect of medicine by following the lucid instructions to be found in *The Physical Examination*. The reader of this book will be fully rewarded.

Robert B. Greenblatt, MD
Professor Emeritus of Endocrinology
Medical College of Georgia
Honorary Fellow – American Academy of Family Physicians

Preface to the Dutch edition

The idea of writing this book coincided almost exactly with the establishment of a 'skills laboratory' of the Medical School in the University of Limburg. The basic concept was (and is) that the acquisition of medical skills should occur with the least possible dependence on teachers and patients. Therefore, we had to find a way independent of teachers to convey to students as exactly as possible how a given examination should be done. The method, described step-by-step, proved to be extremely helpful and highly valued.

It is unusual for a general practitioner to write a book of this kind, but not illogical. The physical examination in all its aspects is part of the daily work of the general practitioner. He has therefore acquired a great deal of experience with, and facility in the basic skills pertaining to the fields of medicine, orthopaedics, neurology, otorhinolaryngology, and ophthalmology. This text, after consultation of the literature, was submitted for comment to another general practitioner, a specialist, a medical student, and the skills instructors (most of them nurses). Their comments contributed greatly to the development of the text. During this process we were struck by the number of ways there are to perform a given examination; the choice of method is often arbitrary. The preference for standardization can be justified on the following grounds:

1. It is not inconceivable that at present the same examination performed by three doctors would yield three different sets of results, mainly because each of them used his own, divergent method.

2. A uniform approach would strongly promote the mutual acceptability and accuracy of the examination results.

3. It would be highly advisable to give students a chance to acquire familiarity with a well thought out and soundly motivated method of examination − instead of giving them a superficial acquaintance with five or six 'fashions' and proficiency in none of them.

Lastly, experience with, and belief in, a particular method form the basis for a well executed examination. The methods I have described here should be read in that sense.

Critical analysis of the available standard works shows that they share one shortcoming: none of them is systematic. I chose a site-orientated classification because physical examinations are often complaint-orientated and complaints are often site-related. For the individual organ I have given preference to a division into aspects of each examination, performed separately in common situations and to a sequence commonly used. It cannot be denied, in any case, that classification according to examination method (inspection, percussion, palpation, and the like) is highly artificial and inconvenient.

The reader may find it a drawback that pathophysiological backgrounds, interpretations of results, and differential-diagnostic considerations are not dealt with. I think there is more than enough good material available, and have therefore included little of this kind of information. Where it seemed useful, brief explanations indicated by a large dot (•) are given.

I hope that students and general practitioners will have as much pleasure in using this book as I have had in writing it. Perhaps the reader now has the opportunity to become better trained than was once possible at the bedside, and perhaps the general practitioner will find that after many years of routine work some of the sharp edges of his examination techniques have become dulled. I hope that they, like myself, will notice that even the techniques they have used daily in their practice can be improved.

L. Lodewick
Maastricht, 1978

Contents

A   Basic skills

1 The technique of inspection

Purpose
To describe some aspects of great importance to inspection.

Procedure
1 Very good illumination is essential.
  •Natural light is to be preferred.
  Keep in mind that artificial light can obscure some important features (e.g., jaundice).

2 Make sure that the temperature in the examining room is comfortable.

3 Make sure that what you want to inspect is clearly visible. Do not hesitate to ask the patient to take off some or all clothing.

4 If necessary, use a magnifying glass to aid inspection.

5 Always clearly define what you see: try to realize what you are observing, and describe it as accurately as you can.

6 Be especially conscious of your first impression of a patient. Pay particular attention to, for instance, behaviour, expression, general appearance, clothing, posture and movement.

7 Take the time to use your eyes well.

8 Be systematic in your inspection and in describing what you see.

9 When necessary, make a comparison with the opposite side of the patient's body.

A 2   The technique of auscultation

Purpose
To listen to the sounds in the body.

Procedure

The stethoscope

1 Use a binaural stethoscope.

2 Be sure that the ear-pieces fit the external meatus adequately.

3 Use a stethoscope with short tubes (25 – 30 cm).

4 The tubing should have thick walls (1/8th inch (3 mm); Figure 1).

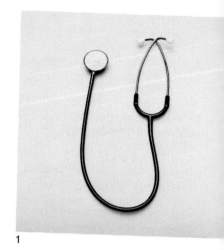

1

5 The internal diameter should be 3 mm.

6 A stethoscope with two tubes is better than one with a branched tube (T-shaped).

7 Use a combination stethoscope providing both a membrane and a cup, preferably rubber rimmed (less cold than bare metal).

8 The membrane should have a diameter of 3.5 – 4 cm (Figure 2).

9 The cup should have a diameter of 3.8 cm and a volume of 6.2 cm^3 (Figure 3).

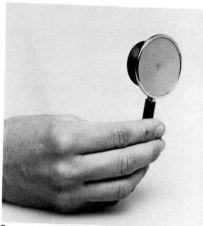

2

Use of the stethoscope

1 Perform the examination in a quiet and restful examining room.

2 In particular, there must be no low-frequency sounds in or penetrating the room.

3 Make certain that the temperature in the room is high enough: in a patient who is chilled or shivering, the tremor of the deep muscles will be audible.
 • Examination of the thoracic region is performed most comfortably with the patient in the semi-reclining position.

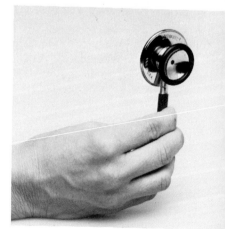

3

4 Place the ear-pieces in your ears
(Figure 4).

5 Make certain that your ears are thus
well plugged, but without unpleasant
pressure.

6 Make certain that the longitudinal axes
of the external meatus and that of the
ear-pieces coincide.

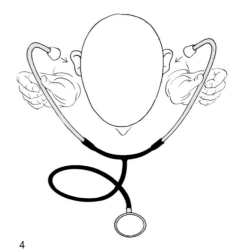

4

7 Select the cup or the membrane
according to what you want to hear.
  ● The cup transmits mainly low-frequency
  sounds.
  ● The membrane filters out the low-
  frequency sounds, and one thus hears
  mainly the high frequencies.

8 By varying the pressure with which you
apply the cup to the skin, you can
regulate the frequency filtration.
  ● Under low pressure mainly low
  frequencies are audible and under
  strong pressure mainly high frequencies.
  ● Low-frequency tones include:
  - presystolic murmurs
  - diastolic murmurs
  - auricular tones
  - 1st, 2nd and 3rd heart sounds
  - gallop rhythm
  - fetal heart sounds
  ● High-frequency sounds include:
  - systolic murmurs
  - pericardial friction

9 Hold the cup or membrane not by the
covered rim but by the metal part, so
that any static electricity is discharged.

A 3　The technique of percussion

Purpose
To delineate the margins of organs or parts of organs differing in air content, by means of indirect finger—finger percussion.

Procedure
1 The patient removes whatever clothing is necessary.

2 Place the middle (or index) finger of the left hand (for the left-handed use the right hand) firmly and flat on the patient's body (Figure 1).

3 With the bent middle (or index) finger of the other hand, strike a short, sharp blow on the distal phalanx (just below the nail) of the opposite finger. The best effect is obtained with a wrist action (Figures 2 and 3).

4 Define the percussion tone you hear.
● Sonorous percussion tone: a rather low, strongly resonating tone (e.g., given by an air filled lung).
● Dull percussion tone: a muffled, short-lasting sound, not sonorous and not resonating, of limited intensity (given by organs containing no air).
● Tympanic percussion tone: this tone is higher and more resonant than the sonorous type (given by air containing, relatively small hollow organs such as the stomach).

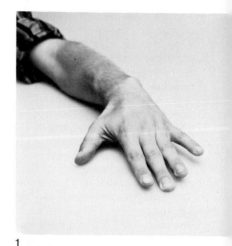

1

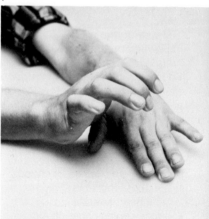

2

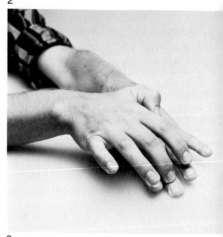

3

4 The technique of palpation

Purpose
To obtain an impression, by feel, of the shape, size, consistency and quality of an organ or structure.

Procedure
- Palpation is usually the last of the diagnostic methods to be applied and is usually preceded by inspection, auscultation, and percussion (which are less disturbing to the patient).

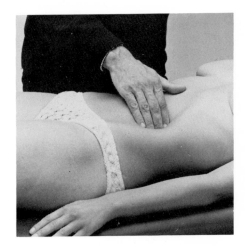

1 The area to be examined should be bare.

2 Make sure your hands are not cold.

3 Always tell the patient what you are about to do.

4 You can in principle palpate with all of your fingers.

5 The index finger and thumb are most sensitive in this respect (ear, page 117; vagina, page 184, and rectum, page 173).

6 Palpation of the abdomen is done with a flat hand and light finger pressure.

7 With the 2nd, 3rd and 4th fingers of either hand close together it is often possible to determine the outline of a structure or organ (see Figure 1).

8 Palpation is also done with both hands.

9 Use your eyes during palpation; pay special attention to the patient's face.

10 Listen carefully during palpation to the patient indicating painful sensations.

11 While palpating an organ, try to describe a number of its characteristics: the size, the shape, the consistency, the surface and the relation to its surrounding organs.

12 Palpate systematically.

13 Always try to define what you think you are feeling.

B   Basic examination

Inspection of the body shape, posture and movement

Purpose
To obtain an impression, by means of inspection, of the build, posture and movement of the patient for the evaluation of the patient's general condition.

Procedure

1 The patient should remove his clothes.

2 Attempt to obtain an impression of the build of the body. Pay special attention to the ratio between the skeleton and soft tissue (muscle development and amount of fat). Form an impression of the proportions of the body as well.

3 Note excessive height or shortness in stature.

4 Note the relationship between the size of the head, the size of the trunk and the length of the extremities (see Figure 1).

5 Try to classify the patient (Asthenic, Athletic, or Pycnic in build).

6 With the patient supine, look for any obvious deformities in body shape.
 • Some patients assume a particular position that is the least uncomfortable for them.

7 Note limitation of movement and also any restriction in normal movement.

8 Note the presence of involuntary movements (e.g. chorea).

9 Have the patient stand and walk. Pay attention to the posture and gait: the manner of walking, swinging of the arms, position of the head, the movement of the legs (firm steps or shuffle) and how fast the patient walks.

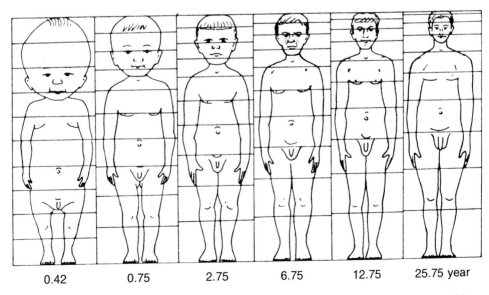

| 0.42 | 0.75 | 2.75 | 6.75 | 12.75 | 25.75 year |

B 2 Inspection of the skin and mucous membranes

Purpose
To obtain an impression of the condition of the skin and mucous membranes by means of inspection.

Procedure
1 Illumination must be very good.

2 Examine the skin and mucous membranes with the naked eye (if necessary, with a magnifying glass).

3 Inspect the skin as a whole; do not limit yourself to local abnormalities.

4 Inspect the hair, nails and mucous membranes thoroughly.

5 When you find skin abnormalities, note the localization, pattern, color, shape, size and margins.

6 Pay particular attention to:
- hair distribution
- thickness, or coarseness of skin
- hardness or callosities
- subcutaneous bleeding, or bruises
- color
- scars
- edema
- scaling
- sweating.

7 While inspecting the mucous membranes pay special attention to:
- secretions
- color
- signs of inflammation
- petechia (pinpoint hemorrhages)
- tumors and nodules
- ulceration
- moistness.

Evaluation of the nutritional and hydration state

Purpose
To obtain an impression of the patient's nutritional and hydration status for the evaluation of the general condition.

Procedure

A The nutritional state

1 The patient should undress.

2 Inspect the patient's skin.
 ● An infant has an appreciable subcutaneous layer of fat, and this gives the body rounded lines.

3 Note whether the skin is loose or flaccid.

4 Pay special attention to the eye sockets, abdomen, and cheeks.
 ● In serious sickness all three are sunken.

5 Evaluate the hair:
 - Is it falling out?
 - Does it have a healthy shine?

6 Combine this impression with others (e.g., the skull's fontanelles, the moistness of the mucous membranes, skin turgor and weight).

7 If appropriate, measure the thickness of skin folds.

B The hydration state

1 Ask the patient to stick out his tongue.

2 Inspect the tongue and mucous membranes to see if they are dry or moist.

3 Ask about the frequency of urination.

4 Combine these findings with others (e.g., nutritional status, fontanelles, sunken eyes if present, skin color, level of consciousness, skin temperature, color and specific gravity of the urine).

5 Obtain information about fever, perspiration, thirst, fluid intake.

6 Evaluate turgor:
   - examine the skin of the abdomen or upper leg;
   - take a fold of skin between your thumb and index finger, lift this fold and rotate it 90° (see Figure 1), estimate the rate at which the fold disappears as a measure of dehydration.
   • Normally, such a fold disappears rapidly.
   - Examine for the presence of edema; pay special attention to the sacral region (especially in patients confined to bed), the ankles, lower legs and orbital area.
   • When the patient has pitting edema, a pressure mark left by a finger remains visible for some time after the pressure has been released (Figure 2).

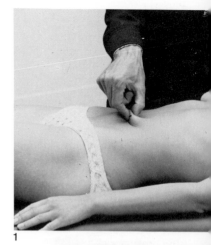

1

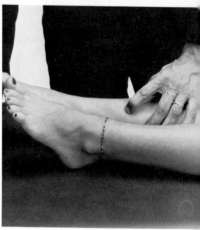

2

Palpation of the skin

Purpose
To obtain an impression of the condition of the skin as an organ, and the local condition of the various parts of the skin by palpation.

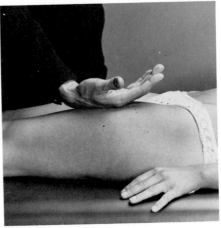

1

Procedure

1 Palpate according to the general method (A4).

2 During palpation of the skin, pay special attention to:
- the temperature of the skin (use the back of the hand; see Figure 1),
- the elasticity of the skin,
- the turgor of the skin,
- the degree of moistness or dryness,
- the presence of scaling,
- the presence of edema (pitting edema and constant edema),
- the presence of nodules (within, on, or below the skin's surface): note the size, shape, consistency, and relationship with the surrounding tissue.

B 5   Evaluation of the pulse

Purpose
To obtain an impression of the quality of the radial pulse.

Procedure

1 The patient should be sitting or lying down and relaxed.

2 The arm is relaxed; jewelry etc. has been removed.

3 Feel the pulse:
 - Find the radial artery (Figure 1).
 - Feel the pulse with the tips of the 2nd, 3rd and 4th fingers of the right or left hand. From the radial side, take hold of the lower arm just above the wrist, your thumb lying dorsally and the finger tips on the palmar surface of the wrist (Figures 2 and 3).

4 First attempt to obtain an impression of the condition of the wall of the vessel.
 • Normally, this is hardly palpable; the margins are indistinct, the vessel flattens easily under pressure and is highly elastic.

5 Next attempt to obtain an impression of the pulse beat.

6 Estimate the rate of the beat first.

7 Note whether the rate is constant or variable.

8 Then note the intensity of the pulse beat (e.g., strong, bounding, feeble or weak).

9 Evaluate the regularity of the pulse.

10 Lastly, count the number of beats per minute.

11 For this purpose, count the beats you feel within 30 seconds.

12 Record the number of beats per minute.

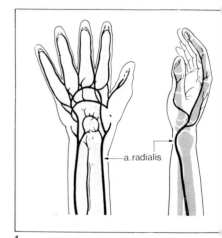

a. radialis

1

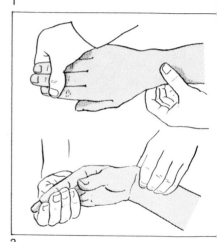

2

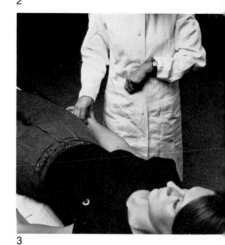

3

B 6   Measurement of the blood pressure

Purpose
Measurement of blood pressure as an estimate of cardiovascular function.

Procedure
1 Sit down opposite the patient.

2 Explain what you are about to do.

3 Expose the left arm of the seated or supine patient (wristwatch removed).

4 Ask the patient to place the forearm on the table or by his side on the couch and to relax.

5 Make sure there is no compression of the upper arm by clothing.

6 Use a mercury sphygmomanometer (Figure 1).

7 Wrap the cuff comfortably but closely fitting (not tightly) around the left upper arm about 5 cm above the elbow fold (Figures 2–4).
- 12 cm cuff for adults,
  14 cm cuff for arm circumferences > 35 cm,
  6–8 cm cuff for children,
  2.5 cm cuff for children < 1 year.

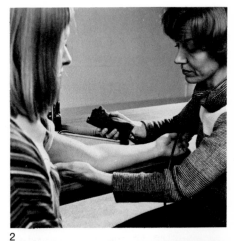

1

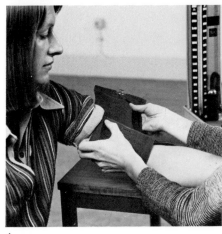

2

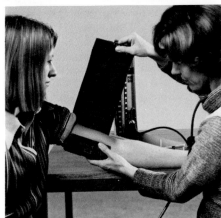

3

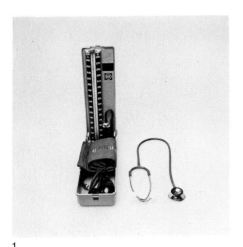

4

8 Controleer de nulstand (afb. 5).

9 Pomp de meter snel op tot 220 mm Hg (afb. 6).

10 Controleer, of de a.radialis niet meer pulseert (i.v.m. de z.g. 'silent gap'; afb. 7).

11 Verzoek de patiënt pompbewegingen met de hand te maken (afb. 8 en 9).

12 Draai het ventiel voorzichtig open en laat de kwikkolom 2 - 3 mm/sec. dalen.

13 Plaats de stethoscoop in de elleboog-holte ter plaatse van de a.brachialis. Gebruik het membraan van de stethoscoop (afb. 10).
   • Wanneer u de eerste tonen hoort, noteert u de op dat moment op de kolom aangegeven waarde als systolische tensie. Wanneer de tonen geheel wegvallen noteert u de op dat moment op de kolom aangegeven waarde als diastolische tensie.

14 Laat de manometer teruglopen tot 0 mm Hg.

15 Meet de bloeddruk nog een tweede maal.

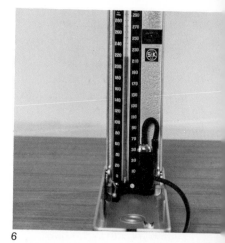

6

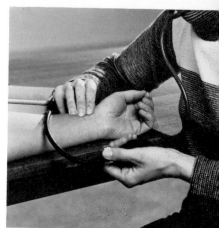

7

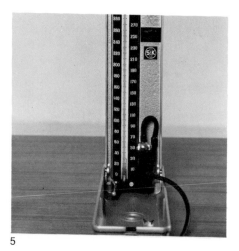

5

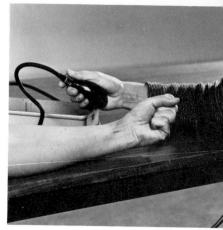

8

Errata for page 18.

8 Check that the reading on the sphygmomanometer is zero before inflating the cuff.

9 Pump the meter up rapidly to 220 mmHg (Figure 6).

10 Check whether the radial artery lacks pulsation (Figure 7).

11 Ask the patient to make pumping movements with the fist (Figures 8 and 9).

12 Open the valve carefully and allow the mercury column to drop 2–3 mm/second.

13 Place the stethoscope in the hollow of the elbow above the brachial artery. Use the membrane of the stethoscope (Figure 10). Listen for the onset of sounds and the disappearance of sounds as the manometer level drops.

14 Allow the manometer to drop to 0 mmHg.

15 Measure the blood pressure a second time.

16 Remove the cuff (Figure 11).

17 Note both readings as a fraction; round off downward to the nearest even number.

18 If the difference between the first and second measurement is > 10 for the systolic and > 5 mmHg for the diastolic pressure, note as the definitive pressure the highest systolic value and the associated diastolic value. If the differences are larger, the measurement should be repeated for a third time after 30 minutes rest.
   •A pressure of < 140/90 is normal.

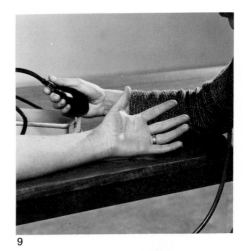

9

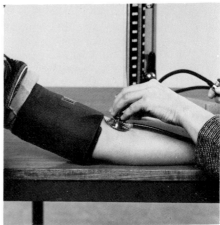

10

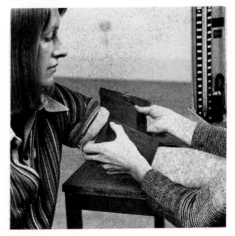

11

B 7   Evaluation of respiration

Purpose
To obtain an impression of the
respiratory function by inspection.

Procedure
1 Ask the patient to expose the upper part
of the body.

2 Note the thoracic and abdominal
respiratory movements.

3 First attempt to form an impression of
the quality of the respiration.

4 Do this by close observation (without
making the patient conscious that you
are doing so).

5 In many cases palpation (with the flat
hand) can provide considerable
information, especially by comparison
of the two sides (Figure 1).

6 At inspiration, pay special attention to
(see also Figures 2 and 3):
   - the sideways movement of the thorax,
   - the widening of the epigastric angle,
   - the increase of the antero−posterior
   width of the thorax,
   - the increase of the abdominal curve,
   forward.

7 At exhalation, pay special attention to:
   - the sinking back of the ribs,
   - the narrowing of the epigastric angle,
   - the reduction of the antero−posterior
   width of the thorax,
   - the decrease in the abdominal curve,
   inward.

8 Note:
   - the duration of inspiration and
   exhalation,
   - the regularity of the respiration,
   - the depth of the respiration,
   - the symmetry of the two halves of the
   thorax,
   - local anomalies during respiratory
   movement,
   - chest and abdominal respiration,
   - retraction of the intercostal spaces.

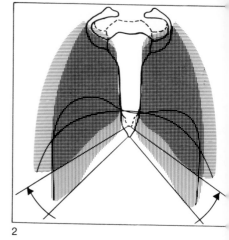

1

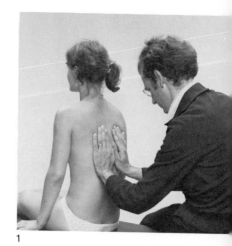

2

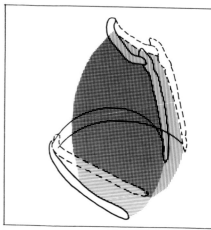

3

9 Also pay attention to:
   - the use of any auxiliary respiratory
     muscles, e.g., those of the nostrils
     and neck or any cyanosis (central or
     peripheral),
   - the patient's posture (e.g., the typical
     posture during asthma attacks;
     Figure 4).

10 Count the number of respirations per
   minute.

11 Start counting with an inspiration.

12 Count only inspirations.

13 Count for 30 seconds.

14 Record the number of respirations per
   minute.

15 If appropriate, measure the chest
   circumference (D 7.4).

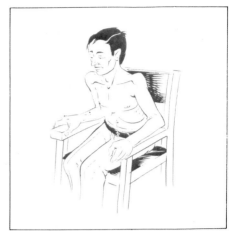

4

Purpose
To determine the height and weight of an adult.

Procedure

A The height

1 Ask the patient to remove his shoes.

2 Stand the patient with the heels against the wall and the feet together.

3 Check that he or she is standing straight and upright against the wall.

4 Press the measuring bar against the head and ask the patient to slip out from under it (Figure 1).

5 Read the height and record it in centimeters.

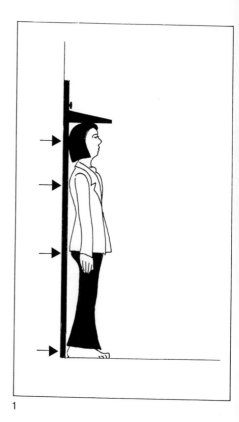

1

B The weight

For normal measurement
Have the patient stand on the scale wearing the same amount of clothing each time, and record the weight in kilograms.

For exact measurement
1 Ask the patient to undress.

2 Check whether the scale is in balance (with the weights in the zero position, the pointer should lie at exactly 0 kg; Figure 2).

3 Lock the scale mechanism.

4 Set the weights at the estimated weight.

5 Ask the patient to mount the scale.

6 Release the mechanism.

7 Bring the scale into balance by moving the sliding weights (Figure 3).

8 Lock the mechanism.

9 Help the patient off the scale.

10 Record the weight in kilograms.

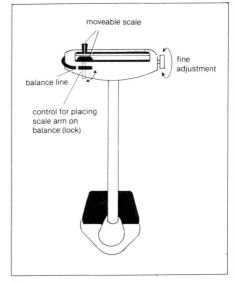

moveable scale

fine adjustment

balance line

control for placing scale arm on balance (lock)

2

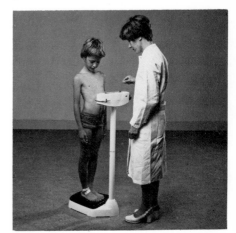

3

B 9　Measurement of length and weight of an infant

Purpose
To determine the length and exact weight of an infant.

Procedure

A The length

1　Lay the child with bare head and feet on the measurement scale.

2　Place its head against the vertical edge.

3　Stretch the child out: it should lie flat and the knees, hips and neck should not be flexed.

4　Move the sliding foot-end against the sole of one foot (Figure 1).

5　Read the length to an accuracy of 0.1 cm.

6　Record the length.

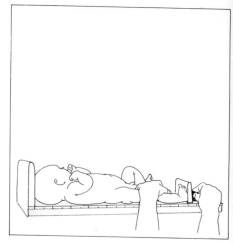

1

●Median normal values (cm)

age (in yr.)	boys	girls
at birth	51.8	50.8
1	77.0	75.6
2	88.9	87.7

B The weight

1 The child should be undressed.

2 Check that the scale is in balance.

3 Make sure the scale tray is warm and lay a thin paper sheet in it.

4 Lock the mechanism.

5 Place the weights at the estimated weight.

6 Lay the child on its back in the scale tray (Figure 2).

7 Release the lock mechanism.

8 Bring the scale into balance by moving the sliding weights.

9 Lock the mechanism.

10 Remove the child from the tray.

11 Read the weight to an accuracy of 5 gram.

12 Note the weight on a graph of weight curves (percentiles).

13 Measure the weight:
   - of a newborn daily,
   - of an infant monthly,
   - of a toddler every 6 months (on a normal scale),
   - of a schoolchild once a year (on a normal scale).

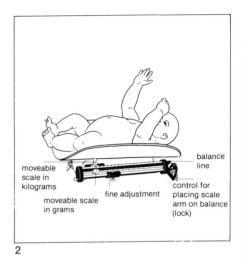

2

● Median normal values (kg)

age (in yr.)	boys	girls
1	3.5	3.4
2	10.5	10.0
3	13.3	12.8

B 10 Measurement of the body temperature rectally

Purpose

To establish the basic body temperature by measurement of the rectal temperature (e.g. in severe fevers or in suspected hypothermia).

Procedure

1 Use a special rectal thermometer with a higher maximum and lower minimum scale than the standard clinical thermometer.

2 Use a lubricating jelly if necessary.

3 The patient lies down on one side with the knees slightly bent.

4 Check the thermometer; if necessary, shake until the mercury column is below 95°F.

5 Place the thermometer in the anus and hold it parallel to the spinal column; if necessary spread the buttocks (Figures 1 and 2).

6 Insert the thermometer into the rectum until the mercury reservoir lies behind the sphincter.

7 Leave the thermometer in place for 3 minutes.

8 Read in degrees Fahrenheit to an accuracy of 0.2°F.

9 Shake the thermometer down.

10 Sterilize the thermometer.

11 Wash your hands.

12 Record the reading.

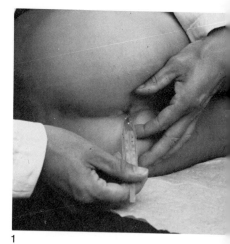

1

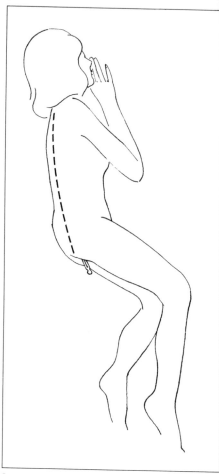

2

C Examination of the nervous system

C 1   Various aspects

Purpose
To obtain an impression of a patient's condition in order to exclude or detect symptoms indicating a disease of the central nervous system or psychological disorders.

Procedure
1 Evaluate:
    - the level of awareness of the patient by the mental function (memory, concentration, intelligence, by way of conversation and any evidence of partial defects),
    - the demeanor and behavior,
    - the speech.
    • The introductions preceding a consultation or physical examination can provide a large amount of information.

2 Check the twelve cerebral nerves.

3 Have the patient undress.

4 Examine the upper extremities.

5 Examine the lower extremities.

6 Examine the trunk.

7 Make notes on your findings.
    • Do not leave the patient unclothed longer than necessary.

The level of consciousness

Attempt to obtain an impression of the patient's level of consciousness.
- In increasing degree of disturbance:
  - somnolent but rousable by calling;
  - stuporous, rousable by calling but not always reacting adequately;
  - rousable by powerful shaking but not by voice;
  - absence of any adequate response to noise or passive movement;
  - reaction to pain stimuli by purposeful defence;
  - reaction to pain stimuli with random response;
  - no reaction, even to strong pain stimuli.

The psychological function

1 Short-term memory: evaluate *response* (ask the patient to repeat a four figure number in reverse or a five figure number in the same sequence); evaluate *retention* (ask the patient to repeat a five figure number after a 15 minute interval); evaluate *reproduction* (ask the patient to repeat a story).

2 Medium-term memory: ask the patient to tell what he or she had for meals the day before or saw on TV.

3 Long-term memory: ask the patient to tell about the past; biographical gaps are particularly important.

4 Concentration: have the patient recite the months of the year in reverse order.

5 Intelligence: ask the patient about his or her educational level and age of finishing school; pay attention to extent of vocabulary.

6 Note partial defects: inability to read, write, count, remember or complete a simple questionnaire or form correctly.

Other assessments

Does the patient express emotions by mimicry or pantomime?

Behaviour patterns

Note such features as facial tics, eye contact, nose picking, wriggling or fidgeting. Is the patient's behavior childish, anxious, tense, euphoric, depressive?

Speech

1 Consider the patient's voice: Is it nasal, hoarse, or clipped? Is the voice clear, high or low? Does it sound monotonous or melodious?

2 Then note the use of language: Try to assess the extent of the vocabulary. Does the individual talk coherently? Is there a tendency to digress?
 • Use of language is strongly determined by intelligence and educational level.

3 Note the articulation. Distinguish between lisping, slurring of words, mumbling. Is the patient a slow or fast talker?

4 In children, watch for retarded speech development.
 • A 4-year-old should be able to articulate normally.
 • Retarded speech development is often due to poor hearing.
 • The most common speech defects are lisping and stuttering.

5 In an aphasic patient, attempt to distinguish between motor and sensory aphasia.
 • Remember that in a patient with aphasia the intelligence is usually not affected.
 • Most aphasic cases are motor or a combination of motor and sensory disturbances.

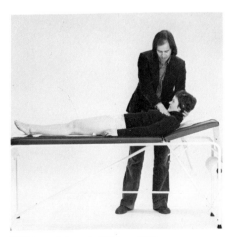

1 The neck is not stiff (see C 2)

C 2   Signs of meningitis

Purpose
To detect signs that could indicate that the meninges are in an inflamed condition.

Procedure
1 Meningitis: resistance and pain when the head is bent forwards but not when it is turned (Figure 1). Opisthotonus is sometimes present.
  • Stiff neck: pain and resistance on forward bending and turning of the head.

2 Kernig's sign: raising of stretched leg produces flexion of hip and knee joints (Figure 2).

3 Brudzinski's sign I: forward bending of the neck produces flexure movements in both legs (Figure 3).

4 Brudzinski's sign II: maximal flexure of hip and knee joints of one leg produces flexure movements in the hip and knee of the other leg (Figures 4 and 5).

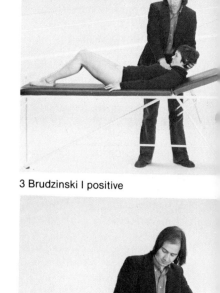

3 Brudzinski I positive

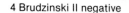

4 Brudzinski II negative

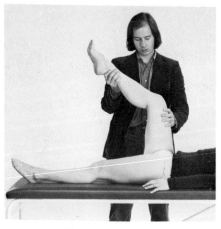

2 Kernig positive

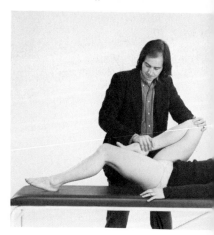

5 Brudzinski II positive

C 3 The twelve cranial nerves

C 3.1 Olfactory and Optic nerve

Olfactory nerve

1 The patient should be seated with mouth and eyes closed.

2 Check that the nasal passages are patent and unblocked.

3 Test each nostril separately (Figure 1).
   - Special substances are available to test the sense of smell (powdered coffee, nutmeg, pepper).

4 Use these if the patient cannot smell coffee.
   - Inability to smell H_2S indicates anosmia.
   - Inability to smell ammonia (function of trigeminal nerve) suggests that the anosmia is probably psychogenic.

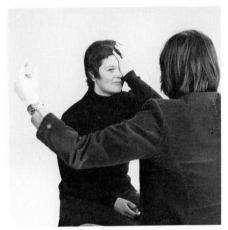
1

Optic nerve

1 Assess vision of each eye separately with the letter chart (see D 2-10).

2 Determine the visual field for both eyes separately:
   - sit straight in front of the patient at a distance of a metre,
   - test each eye with the other shielded (Figure 2),
   - ask the patient to look at your nose,
   - with the fingers moving, bring your hands from the side to the centre or up and down and then in the reverse direction (Figure 3),
   - ask the patient to say when he sees the moving fingers.
   - This test gives a rough impression of the field of vision.
   - You can to some extent compare the patient's field of vision with your own by closing one eye and noting when you see the moving fingers.

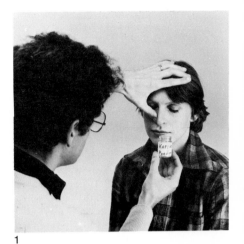
2

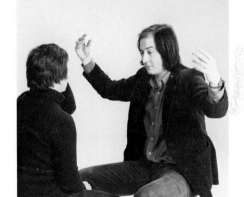
3

C 3.2 Oculomotor nerve, Trochlear nerve and the Abducens

A The pupils

Inspection
1 Note the shape: is the pupil round?

2 Note the width of the pupil (miosis, mydriasis).

3 Are the pupils the same size?

Function
1 Reaction to light (Figures 1 and 2):
   - shield one eye,
   - expose the pupil of the other to a strong light suddenly,
   - observe whether the pupil of that eye becomes smaller,
   - after that, examine the other eye to see whether it shows the same behavior.

2 The convergence reaction (perform only if the reaction to light is absent):
   - ask the patient to look at an object held at a distance of 2 meters,
   - move the object slowly toward the patient's nose,
   - ask the patient to continue looking at the object,
   - note whether the pupil contractions are equal.

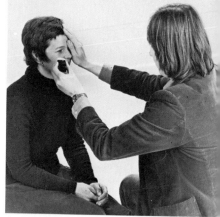

1

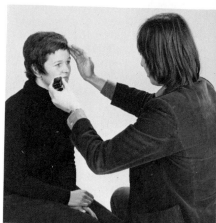

2

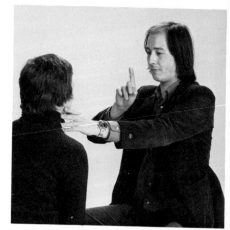

3

B The eye muscles (Figures 3–7)

1 Ask the patient to look straight ahead:
   - are the eyes in parallel or is there convergent or divergent strabismus?
   - does the patient complain of double vision?

2 Ask the patient to look:
   - to the right,
   - to the left,
   - upward to the right,
   - upward to the left,
   - downward to the right,
   - downward to the left.

3 Attempt a double-vision analysis (Figure 8).

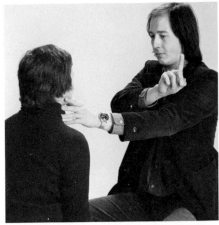

6

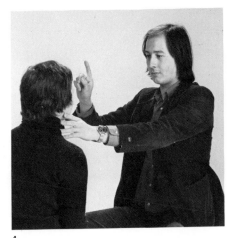

4

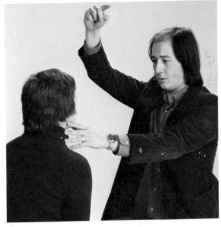

7

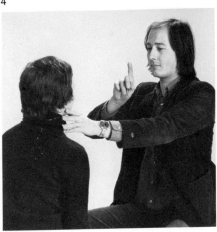

5

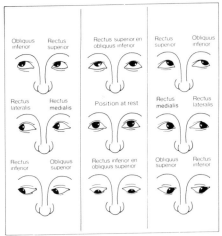

8

35

C 3.3   Trigeminal nerve

A Sensitivity

The corneal reflex

1 The patient should be sitting or lying down.

2 If contact lenses are used, they should be removed.

3 Touch the cornea with the tip of an applicator (e.g. cotton wool bud).

4 Make certain that you do not touch the eyelashes.

5 Make certain that the patient does not see the applicator (approach from the side).
   - If the patient blinks, the corneal reflex is intact (positive).
   - If the patient does not react, the corneal reflex is absent.

6 Compare the right and left eyes.

The facial skin

1 Test the sensitivity of the facial skin at three levels: the chin, the nose and the forehead (Figures 2–4).

2 Test the sensitivity with an applicator, a needle or your fingers.

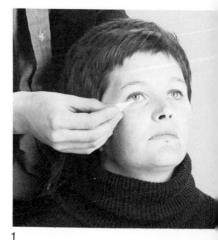

3

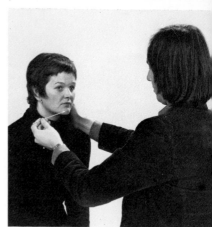

2

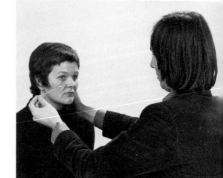

1

B Motor function

The masseter reflex

1 Stand in front of the patient.

2 With your index finger, tap the patient's chin (Figure 5).
 • A positive (i.e. normal) reflex is a contraction of the masseter muscle.

3 You can also percuss the patient's chin indirectly: place the tip of your left index finger on the patient's chin and tap it with your other index finger.
 • A masseter reflex is pathological if the contraction of the muscle is strongly increased.

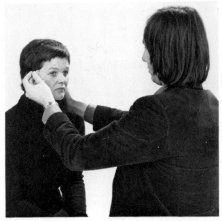

4

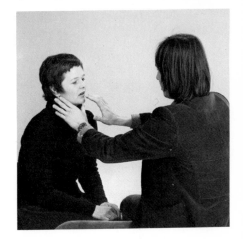

5

37

C 3.4 Facial nerve and Vestibulo-cochlear nerve

Facial nerve

A Sensitivity

1 Test the sense of taste (anterior two-thirds of the tongue) with:
   - a 20% sugar solution,
   - a 10% saline solution,
   - a 5% citric acid solution, and
   - a 1% quinine solution.

   Make certain that the patient keeps the tongue extended until the substance has been identified.

   Make certain that the patient's nostrils are completely closed off.

   Test both the right and left halves of the tongue.

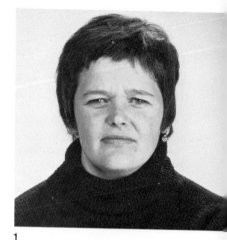

1

B Motor function

1 Have the patient do the following:
   - frown (Figure 1),
   - raise the eyebrows,
   - close the eyes,
   - wrinkle the nose,
   - whistle (Figure 2),
   - show the teeth,
   - laugh (Figure 3),
   - expand the cheeks.

2 Evaluate the symmetry at rest.

3 Compare the right and left sides of the face at each step.

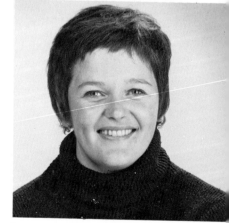

2

4 Perform the tear formation test:
   - using a solution to anesthetize the conjunctivae,
   - insert a piece of filter paper (5 cm long and 0.5 cm wide) in the conjunctival sac,
   - fold the filter paper such that it hangs downward,
   - after 5 minutes, see whether the paper has become moist, and if so how far (Figure 6).
   - Normally, at least 3 cm has become moist after 5 minutes.

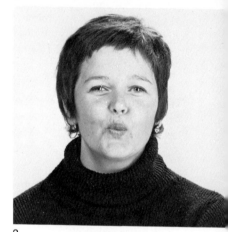

3

Vestibulo-cochlear nerve

1 Evaluate the hearing (D 5.5).

2 When hearing is impaired, distinguish
   between conduction and perceptive
   deafness (see D 5.7).

3 Check for absence of dizziness:
   - differentiate between (e.g.) light-
     headedness and vertigo.
   ●Dizziness is a subjective phenomenon.

4 Check for disturbances of balance:
   - ask the patient to walk along a straight
     line with the eyes closed (Figure 4).

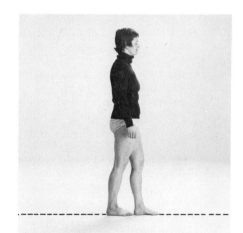

4

5 Check for walking anomalies:
   - ask the patient to walk with his eyes
     open, and evaluate the gait,
   - ask the patient to close the eyes and
     take two steps forward and two steps
     backward a number of times in
     succession.
   ●When anomalies are present the steps
     are taken in a star-shaped pattern,
     because the patient cannot keep to one
     direction. Next:
   - ask the patient to close the eyes,
   - ask the patient to walk on the spot,
     raising the knees high, and after 50
     steps check the amount of turning
     (Figure 5).
   ●45 degrees is acceptable, not more.

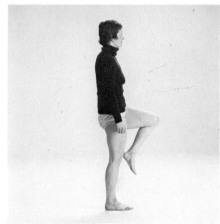

5

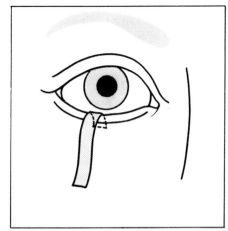

6

39

6 Check for the presence of nystagmus:
   - with the patient at a distance of 1½ metres, ask the patient to look at your finger,
   - move your finger in all directions up to 40 degrees from the midline,
   - estimate the nature and severity of the nystagmus; describe:
     the frequency (rapid or slow),
     the amplitude (wide or short),
     the direction (of the rapid phase),
     the degree (first, second or third),
     the duration (days or weeks).

7 Check tendency to fall (Figure 7):
   - ask the patient to:
     close the eyes,
     stretch the arms forward,
     place the feet together,
   - see whether the patient remains upright,
   - note toward which side the patient leans or falls,
   - have the patient do the same with the eyes open.

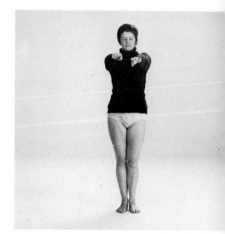

7

3.5 Glossopharyngeal nerve, Vagus nerve, Accessory nerve and Hypoglossal nerve

Glossopharyngeal nerve

1 Test the posterior third of the tongue for taste sensation.

2 Attempt to obtain the gag reflex:
   - ask the patient to open the mouth wide,
   - touch the wall of the pharynx or the soft palate with e.g. an applicator (Figure 1).
   ● A healthy patient will gag.

3 Test the palate's reflex:
   - ask the patient to open the mouth wide,
   - ask the patient to say 'Ah'.
   ● Normally, stimulation of the palate produces a symmetrical and simultaneous upward movement of the palate.

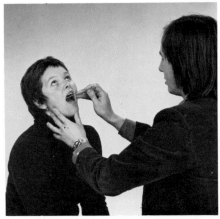

1

Vagus nerve

● Disorders of the recurrent nerve are manifested as hoarseness.

1 You can evaluate or have a specialist evaluate the vocal cords.

Accessory nerve

1 Test the strength of the sternocleido-mastoid muscle.

2 For this purpose, have the patient push your hand away laterally with the head (Figure 2). This tests the sternocleido-mastoid muscle.

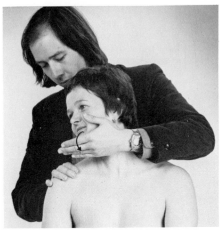

2

3 Compare the power and tone of the sternocleidomastoid muscle on the right and left sides.

4 You can also ask the patient to raise the shoulders. This tests the strength of the trapezius muscle.

Hypoglossal nerve

1 Inspect the patient's tongue, with special attention to atrophy and fasciculation.

2 Have the patient stick out the tongue and move it rapidly from left to right and vice versa.

3 Note anomalies in any direction.

4 Test the strength of the tongue by having the patient push the tongue against the cheek. Assess the strength by palpation.

C 4 Examination of the upper extremity

1 Ask the patient to undress to the waist.

2 Start with a visual evaluation.

3 Pay special attention to any anomalies in muscular development.

4 Involuntary movements.

5 Abnormal posture.

6 Look for contractures.

7 Test for the mobility of the joints (D 11 ff.)

8 Assess the motor function of the arm (C 4.1).

9 Test the sensitivity of the arm (C 4.1).

10 Check a number of arm reflexes (C 4.3).

11 Lastly, perform the coordination tests (C 4.4).

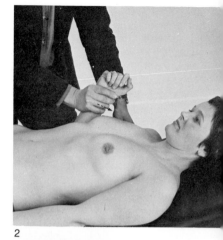

2

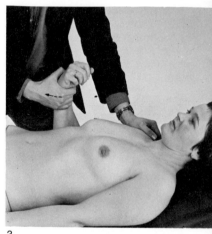

3

Figures 1–7: the motor function and strength tests of the arm (see over)

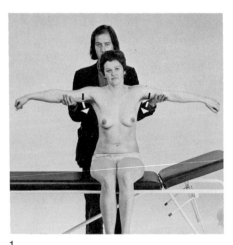

1

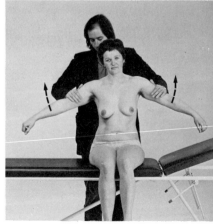

4

4.1 The motor function of the arm

A Muscle tone

1 Ask the sitting patient to relax.

2 Move the elbow and wrist unexpectedly
and rapidly.
- Normally, this movement occurs
smoothly and without resistance.
- In abnormal conditions one encounters
spasticity or the cogwheel phenomenon,
and resistance.

3 Note the presence of contractures.

B Detection of latent paralysis

1 Ask the patient to close the eyes, and

2 stretch the arms out forward with the
palms up and to keep them stretched
(the arms must not touch; see also
Figure 5).
- Normally, the arms can be kept at the
same level for several minutes.

C The strength of the muscles

1 The position test (see above).

2 Estimate the amount of power the
patient can exert in various movements
of the shoulder joint (ab- and adduction,
Figures 1 and 4), the elbow (flexion and
extension, Figures 2 and 3), the wrist
(flexion and extension), and the fingers
(interdigital power and grasping power)
(Figures 6 and 7).

3 At each step compare the right and left
sides.

D Fasciculation

1 Look for involuntary flickering or
movements in the muscles.

E Atrophy

1 Look for atrophy. Measure the
circumference of the arm; pay special
attention to the interosseous muscles
and the muscles of the thumb and little
finger.

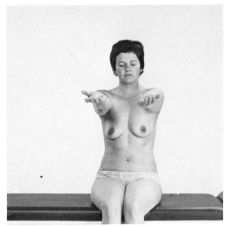

5

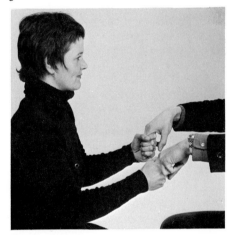

6

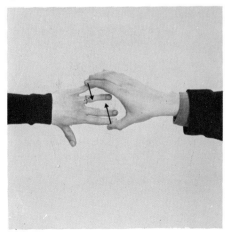

7

C 4.2 The sensations of the arm

A The vital sensations

1 Perception of pain:
   - prick the patient with a needle point or sharp instrument (Figure 1),
   - attempt to determine where this stimulus is felt as a pain stimulus and where it is not.

2 Perception of temperature:
   - test the patient's ability to recognize the warmth or coldness of an object on various parts of the skin.

B The finer sensations

1 Touch (superficial):
   - with a circular movement, stroke the patient's skin lightly with a spatula,
   - try to determine where this is not felt at all or only partially.

2 Discrimination:
   - determine the smallest distance between the points of a compass for which the patient reports feeling two pricks.

3 Vibration:
   - place a vibrating tuning fork on the patient's skin and ask whether the vibrations can be felt in the bone (Figure 2).

4 Shape recognition:
   - have the patient close the eyes and attempt to identify a small object (e.g. a coin or a pen) by touch.

5 Sense of position and movement:
   - the patient's eyes are closed,
   - move his or her fingers with your thumb and index finger,
   - ask the patient to say when a finger is being moved, which finger it is, and which direction it is being moved in (Figure 3).

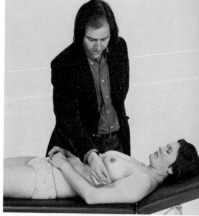

1

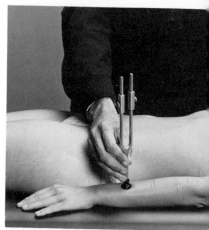

2

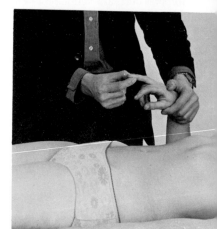

3

4.3 The reflexes of the arm

A The radius reflex

1 The patient should be in the sitting or supine position with one arm slightly bent at the elbow.

2 Bracelets and the like are removed.

3 With the percussion hammer tap lightly and quickly on the styloid process of the radius (Figure 1).
- The hand reacts by adduction due to contraction of the muscles.
- The reflexes can be elevated, normal or absent.

4 Compare the left and right sides.

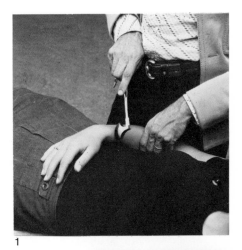

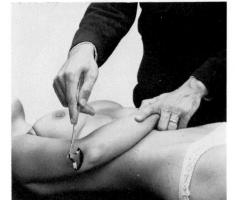

1

B The triceps reflex

1 The patient should be sitting or supine.

2 The arm is relaxed.

3 Stand beside the patient.

4 The arm is bent 90 degrees at the elbow.

5 Tap the tendon of the triceps muscle above the olecranon with the percussion hammer (Figure 2).
- The forearm reacts with slight extension due to contraction of the triceps muscle.

6 Compare left and right and when in doubt repeat the test.
- The reflexes can be elevated, normal or absent.

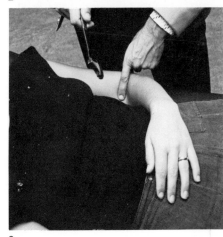

2

C The biceps reflex

1 The patient should be in the sitting or supine position.

2 The arms are relaxed.

3 Stand next to the patient.

4 The arm is bent about 90 degrees at the elbow.

3

5 Place your left index finger in the elbow crease of the left arm on the tendon of the biceps muscle, and tap your index finger with the hammer (Figure 3).

6 Do the same with your thumb on the right arm (Figure 4).
 ● The forearm reacts by lifting slightly due to contraction of the biceps muscle.

7 Compare right and left throughout and repeat the test when in doubt.
 ● The reflexes can be elevated, normal or absent.

D

1 Ask the patient to relax the hand.

2 Lift the patient's middle finger with your middle finger (Figure 5).

3 With the middle finger of your other hand, tap the most distal phalanx of the patient's middle finger.

4 Note whether flexure of the thumb and/or index finger occurs.
 ● Flexion of the thumb indicates a normal reflex.

E

1 Ask the patient to relax the hand.

2 Take hold of the patient's wrist with one of your hands.

3 Take hold of the middle finger of the patient's hand and flex it passively as far as possible at the metacarpophalangeal joint, for extended finger (see Figure 6).

4 Note adduction of the patient's thumb.
 ● This adduction is absent in patients with lesions of the pyramidal tract.

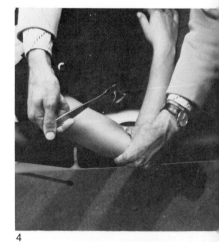

4

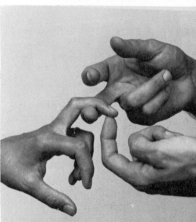

5

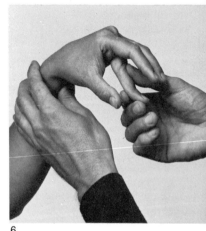

6

1.4 Coordination tests for the arm

A Diadochokinesia

1 Ask the patient to raise both arms sideways and bend them 90 degrees at the elbow.

2 Then ask the patient to perform pro- and supination movements as rapidly as possible (Figure 1).

3 Judge whether this can be done rapidly, and

4 whether it can be done at the same rate on both sides and symmetrically.

B The finger–nose test

1 The patient has the eyes closed and one arm stretched out to the side.

2 Ask the patient to bring first one and then the other index finger to the tip of the nose (Figure 2).

3 Judge:
   - whether the patient can do this, and
   - how it is done (intention tremor, quickly or slowly, or with uncertainty).

C The finger–finger test

1 With the eyes closed, the patient spreads the arms wide.

2 Ask the patient to bring the tips of the index fingers together.

3 Judge:
   - whether the patient can do this, and
   - how it is done (intention tremor, quickly or slowly, or with uncertainty).

D Alternative to the finger–finger test

1 The patient's eyes are closed.

2 Ask the patient to touch your index finger with their own (before the test, the patient is permitted to see where yours is) (Figure 3).

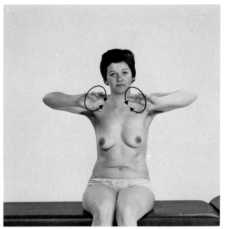

1

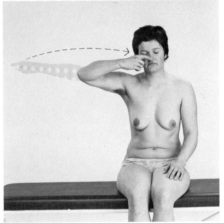

2

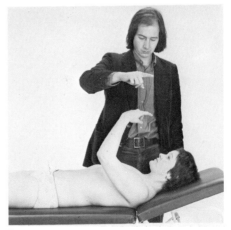

3

3 Judge:
   - whether the patient can do this, and
   - how it is done.

E The rebound phenomenon

1 Ask the patient to bend one elbow while
  you pull in the opposite direction
  (Figure 4).

2 Release the arm suddenly.
  ●Normally, the resulting movement is
  inhibited.

3 Do not forget to protect the patient's
  face in case inhibition of the movement
  does not occur.

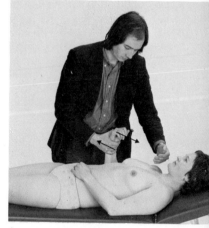

4

5   Examination of the lower extremity

1 Ask the patient to undress below the waist.

2 Start by making a good visual evaluation.

3 Pay special attention to any anomalies in muscle development,

4 involuntary movements,

5 and abnormal posture.

6 Look for contractures.

7 Test the mobility of the joints (D 16 ff.)

8 Examine the motor function of the leg (C 5.1).

9 Test the sensitivity of the leg (C 5.2).

10 Check a number of reflexes (C 5.3).

11 Perform the coordination tests (C 5.4).

C 5.1 The motor function of the leg

A The muscle tone

1 Ask the supine patient to relax. If necessary, distract him or her.

2 Lift the patient's leg suddenly.

3 Note whether this movement occurs easily, smoothly, and without resistance.

4 Compare the right and left sides.

B Detection of latent paralysis

1 The patient should be lying in the supine position with eyes closed.

2 Ask the patient to bend the hips and knees to 90 degrees.

3 Note whether the patient can keep both legs at the same height (Figure 1).

C The power

1 Test the power of the muscles of the upper leg:
   - the patient lies stretched out on the back,
   - press the back of the knees against the table,
   - ask the patient to raise the knees against the pressure of your hand (Figure 2), evaluate the force applied,
   - compare left and right at all stages.
   - Ask the patient to bend the knees,
   - try to restrain the lower leg (Figure 3).
   - Ask the patient to stretch the bent legs,
   - try to restrain the lower leg (Figure 4).

2 Test the power of the muscles of the lower leg:
   - with the patient in the supine position,
   - ask him or her to perform dorsal flexion against pressure exerted by your hands (Figure 5),
   - then ask for the same under a plantar flexion,
   - and lastly, ask for lateral flexion under the same conditions (Figure 6); evaluate the power,
   - compare left and right throughout.

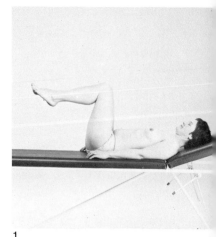

1

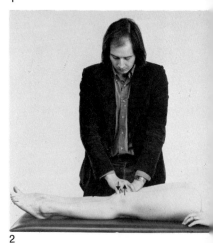

2

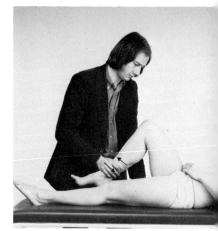

3

D Fasciculation

1 Look for involuntary flickering, or movements of the muscles.

E Atrophy

1 Look for signs of atrophy and measure the circumference of the leg.

F Walking

1 Ask the patient to walk on the toes and then on the heels.

2 Note whether the patient can do this and, if so, how it is done — easily, painfully or with difficulty.

3 Lastly, ask the patient to draw the knee high with each step.

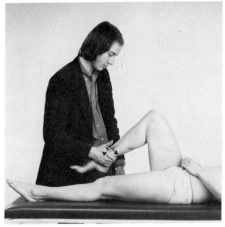

4

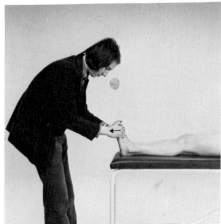

5

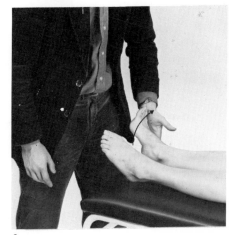

6

C 5.2 The sensations of the leg

A The vital sensations

1 Perception of pain:
   - gently prick the patient's skin with the point of a needle or sharp instrument,
   - try to determine where the patient does and does not feel pain.

2 Perception of temperature:
   - test whether the patient recognizes a cold and a warm object as such, on the various parts of the skin.

B The finer sensations

1 Touch (superficial):
   - with a circular movement, stroke the patient's skin lightly with a spatula,
   - try to determine where this is felt, not felt, or only partially felt.

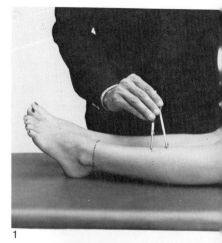

1

2 Discrimination:
   - determine the smallest distance between the points of a compass for which the patient reports feeling two pricks (Figure 1).

3 Vibration:
   - place a vibrating tuning fork on the patient's skin and ask whether the vibrations can be felt in the bone (Figure 2).

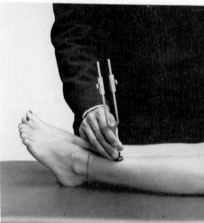

2

4 Sense of position and movement:
   - the patient's eyes are closed,
   - move the toes,
   - ask the patient to say when a toe is being moved, which toe it is, and in which direction it is being moved (Figure 3).

5 Perform finer sensation tests at different levels on the lower limbs.

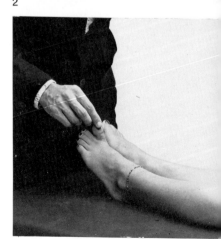

3

C 5.3 The reflexes of the leg

A The knee jerk reflex

1 The patient should be in the (a) sitting or (b) supine position.

2 Make certain that the leg to be examined is as relaxed as possible by
   (a) asking the patient to allow the leg to hang down or to cross the leg to be examined over the other leg;
   (b) supporting the half-bent knee on your left arm.

3 Tap the tendon of the quadriceps muscle just below the patella with the hammer (Figures 1 and 2).
   ●After a short delay there may be an upward movement of the lower leg due to contraction of the quadriceps muscle.

4 If the reflex is difficult to obtain, distract the patient by having him or her hook the hands together, with the fingers flexed, and pulling apart as hard as possible but still keeping the hands together. Percuss while this is being done (Figure 3).
   ●The reflex may be very strong, normal or weak to absent. Rhythmic contraction may also occur.

5 Compare the right and left sides.

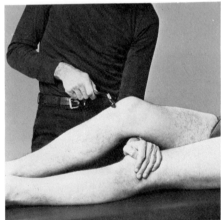

patella

1

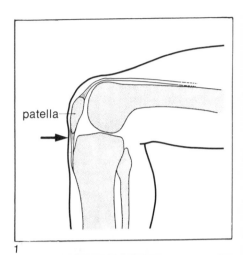

2

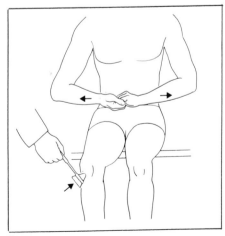

3

B The achilles tendon reflex

1 The patient should kneel on a chair.

2 Ask the patient to relax the lower leg and foot.

3 Tap the achilles tendon with the hammer (Figure 1).
  ● The foot will show plantar flexion due to contraction of the calf muscles.
  ● This reflex can be very strong, enhanced, normal, weakened or absent.

4 Compare the right and left sides.
  ● The following method is used only when the first is not feasible.

5 The patient is supine on the examining table.

6 Bend one of the patient's legs at the knee, while holding the foot firmly.

7 With the hammer in the other hand, tap the achilles tendon (Figure 2).

8 Note the degree of plantar flexion.

9 Compare this reaction with that of the other foot under the same conditions.

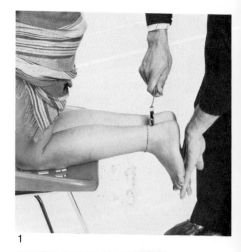

1

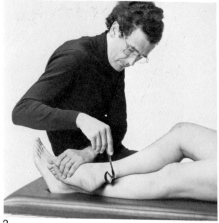

2

C The reflexes of the sole of the foot

1 The patient exposes both feet. Make certain that the feet are warm.

2 Press the lower leg against the table.

3 With the other end of the hammer (or a needle), stroke the lateral edge of the sole of the foot from the heel to the little toe and then over the ball of the foot from the side to the middle (Figure 1).
  - Normally, the big toe (and also possibly the other toes) will show plantar flexion (Figure 2). If the big toe shows a distinct dorsal movement (often accompanied by spreading of the other toes), a pathological reflex (Figure 3) is involved.
  - The foot-sole reflex is often difficult to interpret, because the reaction may be suppressed.

4 If you are in doubt, repeat the test a few times (and if necessary once again later).

5 Compare left and right.

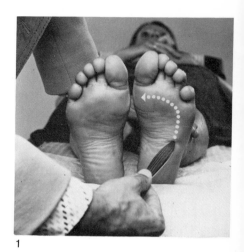

1

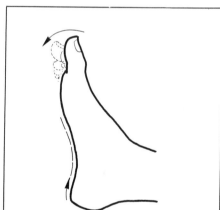

2

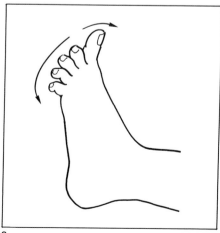

3

C 5.4 Coordination tests for the leg

A The knee–heel test

1 The patient is asked to lie on the back with the eyes closed.

2 Ask the patient to place the heel of one foot on the knee of the other leg.

3 Note whether the patient can do this.

4 Ask the patient to slide the heel down from the knee to the instep of the leg (Figures 1 and 2).

5 Note:
 - whether the patient can do this, and
 - how it is done.

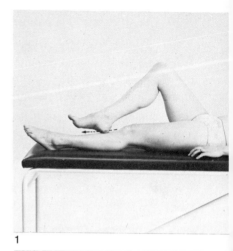

1

B Standing

1 Check whether the patient stands straight, and

2 can remain straight, and

3 can remain straight with closed eyes.

4 Evaluate the patient's posture.

C Walking

1 Ask the patient to walk 'a tightrope' on a straight line.

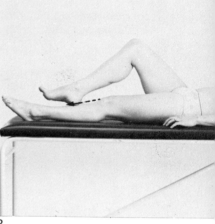

2

C 6   Examination of the trunk

1 Ask the patient to disrobe completely.

2 Start by obtaining a good visual impression.

3 Pay special attention to any abnormalities in muscular development,

4 involuntary movements, and

5 abnormal posture.

6 Check for contractures.

7 Test the mobility of the trunk (D 11).

8 Examine the motor function of the trunk muscles (C 6.1).

9 Test the sensitivity (C 6.2).

10 Check a number of reflexes (C 6.3).

C 6.1 The motor function of the trunk

A The muscle tone

1 Perform a number of back movements
(flexion, extension and rotation)
passively.

2 Try to determine whether these
movements occur easily, smoothly and
without resistance.

B The muscle power

1 Test the strength of the abdominal
muscles:
- with the patient supine,
- ask to have both legs extended and
raised until the heels are about 10 cm
above the examining table (Figure 1),
- see whether the patient can do this,
and how long it can be maintained.
- You can also ask the supine patient to
sit up without using the arms.

2 Test the strength of the back muscles:
- with the patient in the prone position,
- ask him or her to raise the head
(Figure 2).
- You can also ask the patient to pick
something up from the ground,
- and note how this movement is
performed.

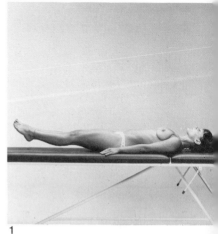

1

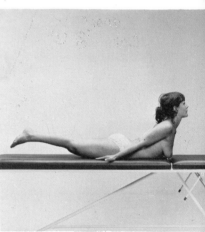

2

C 6.2　The sensations of the trunk

A　The vital sensations

1　Perception of pain:
  - gently prick the patient on the back with the point of a needle or a sharp instrument (Figure 1),
  - try to determine where this is and is not felt as pain.

2　Perception of temperature:
  - test the patient's ability to distinguish between a cold and a warm object at various positions on the skin.

B　The finer sensations

1　Touch (superficial):
  - with a circular motion stroke the patient's skin softly with a spatula (Figure 2),
  - attempt to determine when this is not felt, or not perceived to the same degree.

2　Discrimination:
  - determine the smallest distance between the two points of a compass that the patient still feels as two separate pricks.

3　Vibration:
  - place a vibrating tuning fork on the patient's skin and ask whether the vibration is felt in the bone.

4　Sense of position:
  - take a fold of skin between your thumb and index finger (without causing pain) (Figure 3) or press the patient's skin with a finger,
  - ask the patient to say what he or she feels.

5　Do all of these tests at several positions on the trunk.

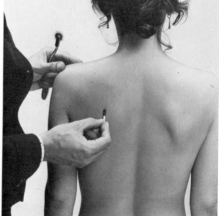

1

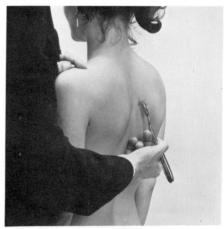

2

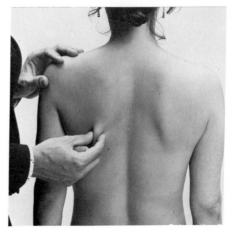

3

C 6.3 Some trunk reflexes

A The abdominal skin reflex

1 The patient should undress and be lying down.

2 Stroke the abdominal skin rapidly and not too hard with a spatula from the side to the middle at three levels (Figures 1 and 2).

3 Note the contractions of the abdominal muscles (degree and symmetry).
 ●In women who have been pregnant and older persons this reflex is often absent or indistinguishable.

B The cremasteric reflex (male)

1 The patient should undress and be lying down.

2 Stroke the skin of the upper leg longitudinally with a spatula.

3 Note contraction of the cremaster muscle (to be evaluated from the contraction of the scrotum and the raising of the testicles).
 ●This reflex is often absent or asymmetrical.

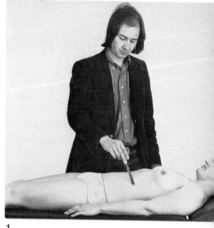

1

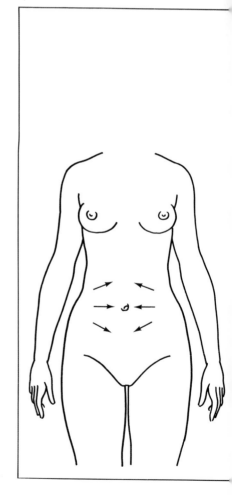

Purpose
To rapidly perform a short neurological examination with little chance that important defects will be missed. (After Prof. T. Murray, Dalhousie University, Halifax, Canada).

Procedure
1 Determine the level of consciousness. Evaluate the psychological function. Pay special attention to the speech.

2 Check the cerebral nerves:
   - perform funduscopy,
   - define the field of vision,
   - examine the pupils, pupil reaction and eye movements, with special attention to nystagmus,
   - test the sensitivity of the face by touching the skin with your fingers,
   - test the facial muscles by asking the patient to close the eyes and laugh,
   - ask the patient to say 'Ah';
   - examine the pharynx and ask the patient to stick out his tongue.

3 Examine the motor functions:
   - test the power of the deltoid, biceps and triceps muscles, the strength of the wrist, and the pinch power of the fingers,
   - look for latent paralysis in the arms and legs,
   - test the power of the hip flexors and knee flexors and extensors,
   - ask the patient to walk on toes and heels,
   - perform finger−nose, diadochokinesia, and knee−heel tests.

4 Test the following reflexes:
   - the biceps and triceps reflexes,
   - the radial muscle reflex,
   - the knee tendon reflex,
   - the achilles tendon reflex,
   - the foot-sole reflex.

5 Evaluate the sensitivity:
   - use a needle to test the skin of the face, shoulder, inside and outside of the upper arm, and the ulnar, medial and radial sides of the hand,
   - test the skin of the thorax, abdomen and thighs,
   - test the skin on both sides of the tibia, the lateral side of the foot and the big toe, and
   - investigate all differences between the left and right sides of the legs. Always prick from distal to proximal.

6 Watch how the patient walks and stands, and ask him to walk along a straight line.

D Examination of separate parts of the body

1 Examination of the head

Purpose
To obtain an impression of the shape and functioning of the head and of a number of the organs it contains.

Procedure
1 The patient may sit or lie down.

2 Ask the patient to remove eye glasses.

3 Start with inspection.

4 Continue with percussion.

5 Then palpate the head.

6 If necessary have X-rays taken and other investigations done.
  • Remember that every head has a front, a back, and two sides and is round.

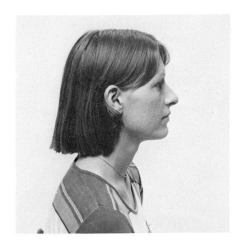

D 1.1 Inspection of the shape of the head

Purpose
To obtain an impression of the shape of the head by inspection.

Procedure
1 Consider the shape of the head.

2 In doing so, try to disregard the hair.

3 Attempt to obtain an impression of the shape of the cranium.

4 Look for any divergence in size or symmetry — the 'steeple' skull and skulls with flat sides, as well as skulls which seem to be too large or too small.

.2 Palpation of the skull (in the baby and the infant)

Purpose
To obtain an impression of the size of the fontanelle — whether bulging or depression is present.

Procedure
1 The child is seated on the lap of the attending adult, or is lying in bed.

2 Palpate the anterior fontanelle.

3 Determine the size of this fontanelle.
  ● The anterior fontanelle has usually closed by the age of 1½ years (at the latest at the age of 2 years).

4 Determine whether the fontanelle shows marked bulging or pressure, or is deeply sunken.
  ● Normally, one sees a very slightly raised fontanelle which usually exhibits some pulsation.

5 Lastly, palpate the various cranial sutures. Note the course, shape and size. (See Figure below.)

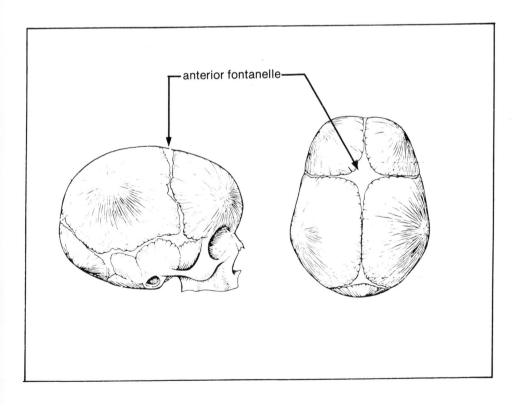

anterior fontanelle

D 1.3 Percussion of the skull

Purpose

To obtain information about any disease processes in the skull by means of percussion.

Procedure

1 Percuss the skull systematically.

2 Listen for changes in the percussion sound (of little diagnostic value).

3 Ask the patient to say whether, and if so where, percussion is painful.

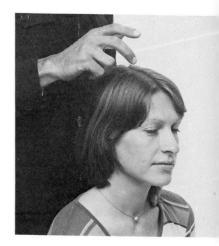

D 1.4 Measurement of the circumference of the skull

Purpose
To measure the cranial circumference.

Procedure
1 The patient should be seated.

2 Measure the circumference of the skull
with a flexible tapemeasure placed on
the fronto-occipital plane.
  • This is the plane through the middle of
the frontal bone and through the upper
side of the occipital bone. Thus, the
largest dimension is measured (Figures
1 and 2).

3 Measure the cranial circumference to an
accuracy of 0.1 cm.

4 Record the cranial circumference in
centimetres.

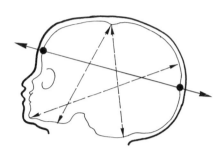

1

• Mean cranial circumference (cm)

age	boys	girls
at birth	34	34
1 month	37.5	36.5
2 months	39.0	38.5
3	40.5	40.0
4	41.5	41.0
5	43.0	42.0
6	44.0	43.0
7	44.0	43.5
8	45.0	44.5
9	45.5	45.0
10	46.0	45.0
11	47.0	45.5
12	47.0	46.0
15	48.0	47.0
18	49.0	47.5
2 years	49.5	48.5
4	50.6	49.6
6	51.4	50.8
8	51.8	51.5
adults	53.8	53.7

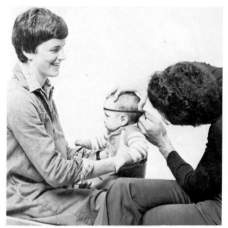

2

D 1.5　Inspection of the scalp

Purpose

To obtain an impression of the quality and quantity of the hair, and the quality of the skin on the head with and without hair, by means of inspection.

Procedure

A The hair-bearing skin on the head

1 Have good illumination.

2 Stand beside or behind the seated patient.

3 Start with inspection of the hair (see Figure 1). Take note of:
   - the amount of hair,
   - the thickness of the hair,
   - the hair line,
   - the color of the hair
   - the dryness or oiliness of the hair,
   - scaling,
   - parasites.

4 Pull out a few hairs and examine the roots under a microscope; note the presence of broken or split hairs.

5 Next, inspect the scalp. For this purpose spread the hair and inspect the entire scalp systematically. Watch in particular for:
   - inflammation,
   - tumors or swellings, e.g. cysts,
   - bald spots,
   - scaling,
   - crust formation,
   - scars,
   - pigmentation or color changes,
   - parasites.

B The hair-free skin of the head

1 Stand in front of the patient and inspect his or her face.

2 Inspect the skin of the neck as well.

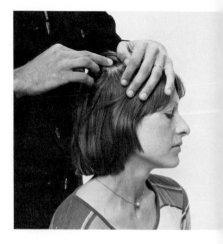

3 Note:
   - inflammation,
   - tumors or swellings,
   - acne,
   - scars,
   - scabs and scaling,
   - color alterations
   - other skin changes.

4 Note changes in the shape of the face edema, "moon" (face or shock).

5 Note the facial color (pale, cyanotic).

6 Note whether the face is symmetrical (facial paresis).

7 Assess the expressivity of the face.

1.6 Palpation of the lymph glands in the neck

Purpose
To obtain an impression of the presence, size and consistency of the lymph glands in the neck.

Procedure
1 The patient has undressed to the waist.

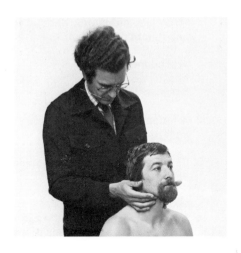

2 The lymph glands in the neck can be found most easily if one stands behind the patient.

3 Palpate systematically.

4 Start in the submental region.

5 Next, palpate the submandibular region.

6 Then palpate the medial triangle.

7 Palpate the sternocleidomastoid muscle and also under it.

8 Pay special attention to the supraclavicular lymph glands.

9 Palpate the lateral triangle.

10 Lastly, palpate the pre- and post-auricular glands.
   - Lymph glands usually remain stationary during swallowing.

11 When you find a lymph gland, note the exact location, shape, size and consistency.

12 Determine the relationship with the surroundings as well (skin, deep tissues and other glands).

13 Do not confuse glands with cysts, if any are present.
   - Cysts are translucent (e.g. branchial cysts).

14 Distinguish between glands and aberrant thyroid gland tissue.
   - Such tissue moves together with the larynx during swallowing.
   - The larger and more firmly fixed a gland is, and the lower its location in the neck, the greater is the chance that it is malignant.

D 2 Examination of the eyes

Purpose
To collect information about the shape
and function of the eye.

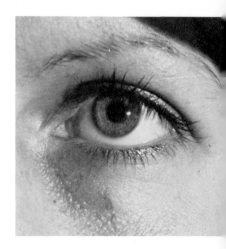

Procedure
1 Provide good lighting, have a good
   portable source.

2 Arrange to be able to examine in the
   dark as well.

3 Explain to the patient what you are
   about to do, be clear when you give
   instructions.

4 Sit (or stand) in front of the patient, this
   position usually facilitates examination.

5 A patient has a right and a left eye.

6 Therefore, compare left and right
   throughout.

7 Keep in mind that the eye is (or should
   be) spherical. Examine from the side,
   from above and from below.

8 The inspection of the eye is most
   important.

9 Assess the various functions of the eye
   (D2.7, 2.8)

10 Perform eye measurements (D2.10).

Inspection of the eyelids

Purpose
To obtain an impression of the shape of
and any anomalies of the eyelids.

Procedure
1 Ask the patient to look straight ahead.

2 Compare the right and left eye.

3 Inspect with the eyes closed as well as
open.

4 Assess the skin of the eyelids and note
any alterations (redness, swelling).

5 Examine the edge of the eyelid
(swelling, crusting, redness).

6 Note the hair growing on the eyelids:
- presence or absence of eyelashes,
- the position of the eyelashes.

7 Also note the extent of the eyelids
opening.

8 Note drooping of the upper eyelid when
the eye is open (ptosis).

D 2.2 Inspection of the conjunctiva

Purpose
To obtain an impression of the condition
of the conjunctiva.

Procedure
1 Ask the patient to look straight ahead.

2 Inspect the conjunctiva; if there is
   redness, determine the kind (superficial
   or deep vascularization), the location
   and the extent.

3 With your thumb draw the lower eyelid
   down (Figure 1).

4 Inspect the conjunctiva and the lower
   conjunctival sac.

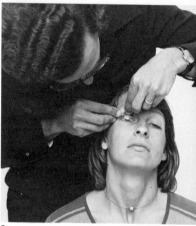

1

5 Look for infections and any pus forming.
   If hyperemia is present, determine
   whether it arises from the conjunctiva or
   deeper lying structures. Determine the
   location and extent of the hyperemia

6 To examine the upper conjunctival sac,
   the upper eyelid must be turned up
   (Figure 2):
   - stand behind the patient,
   - ask the patient to look straight ahead,
   - have a matchstick or something
     similar in one hand,
   - take hold of the eyelashes with the
     thumb and index finger of the other
     hand,
   - draw the eyelid upward, the matchstick
     lying about 1 cm back from the
     eyelashes,
   - use the matchstick as a hinge: the
     eyelid folds back over it and you will
     have a clear view of the conjunctiva.
   - Ask the patient to look downward.
   - When you have finished the
     examination, grasp the eyelashes
     again and draw them forward and
     down to unfold the eyelid.

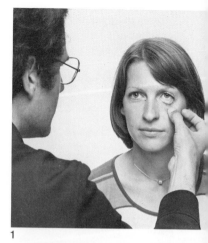

2

7 While inspecting the conjunctiva, examine the deeper-lying sclera as well.

8 In doing so, watch for any redness.

9 Ask the patient to move the eyes as far as possible in all directions, which gives a view of the entire sclera (Figure 3).

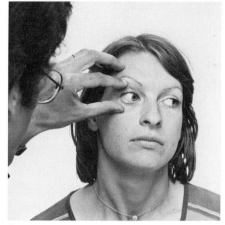

3

D 2.3 The fluorescein test

Purpose
To investigate the cornea by staining
with fluorescein.

Procedure

1 The patient should be seated.

2 Stand behind the patient and ask him to
tip his head backward.

3 Support the patient's head against your
body.

4 Ask the patient to open both eyes and
look at his toes (Figure 1).

5 Explain that you are about to put a drop
of a local anesthetic agent in the eye
(which may sting a little).

6 Add a second drop.
  ●The cornea is now anesthetized.

7 Ask the patient to open one eye.

8 Insert a fluorescein strip under the
upper lid (Figure 2).

9 Ask the patient to close the eye.

10 After 10 seconds remove the strip.

11 Remove excess moisture from the
corner of the eye with an applicator
(with the eye closed, swab from the side
to the medial aspect, not in any other
direction).

12 Illuminate the cornea with a strong light
source (Figure 3).
  ●Lesions of the cornea are then visible
  due to the accumulation of fluorescein.

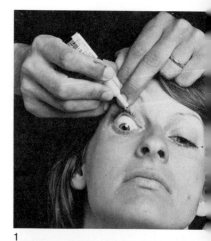

1

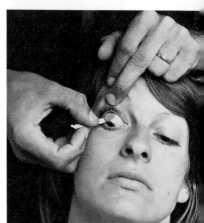

2

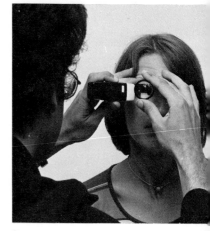

3

Inspection of the cornea

Purpose
To gain an impression of the shape and condition of the cornea.

Procedure
1 View the cornea from the front, above and the side, and note any irregularities of shape.

2 Direct the light over the cornea.
   - With transmitted light the direction of the light beam and the direction in which the eye is looking coincide; for this purpose a normal light source can be used (Figure 1).
   - With reflected light there is an angle between the light source and the line of vision; by preference, a slit lamp is used for this purpose (Figure 2).

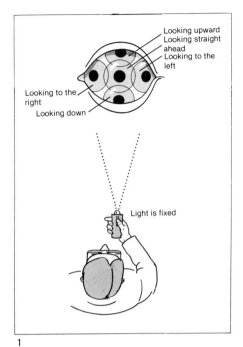

Looking upward
Looking straight ahead
Looking to the left
Looking to the right
Looking down

Light is fixed

1

2

D 2.5   Inspection of the iris and lens

Purpose
To obtain an impression of the shape and function of the iris and the condition of the lens.

Procedure

A The iris

1 Note the color of the iris.

2 Check whether both the pupils are the same size.

3 Check the shape of the pupil.

4 Evaluate the pupil's reaction to light.

5 Check the fluid in the anterior chamber; is it clear?

B The lens

1 Use should always be made of both reflected and transmitted light.

2 The examination should be performed in the dark.

3 Sit down in front of the patient.
  • The best information is obtained when the pupil is dilated.

4 Note the color of the lens under normal transmitted light.
  • Under transmitted light the pupil has a red glow.

5 Check the lens for cloudiness.

6 Move the light source in a circle and examine in its path.

7 Next use reflected light, preferably from a slit lamp.

8 Direct the slit at the eye and check each cross-section thus obtained.

Purpose
To obtain an impression of the retinal
structures by ophthalmoscopy.

Procedure

1 Seat the patient on a chair.

2 Begin by describing what you are about
to do.

3 Apply 1−2 drops of a short-acting pupil
dilating agent, e.g. tropicamide
(Figure 1).

4 Have the room in semi-dark.

5 Sit on a chair directly in front of the
patient (Figure 2).

6 Ask the patient to look about 15° to the
left for funduscopy of the right eye and
about 15° to the right for the left eye.

7 Ask the patient to keep looking at some
point behind you.

8 If the patient wears spectacles remove
them, and remove yours as well if you
wear them.

9 Add up the strength of both sets of
spectacle lenses and set your
ophthalmoscope at this value (Figures 2
and 4).

10 Start the examination with the right eye.

11 Then examine the left eye.

12 Hold the ophthalmoscope as close as
possible to the patient's eye and your
own eye (Figures 3 and 5).

13 Adjust for a sharp image by turning the
ophthalmoscope control.

14 Examine the fundus systematically.

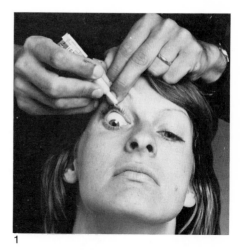

1

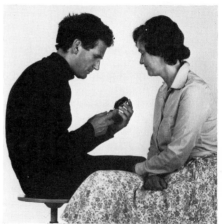

2

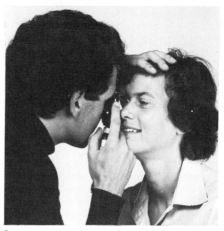

3

15 Follow the large vessels first.

16 Look for stenosis, kinking, and other vascular anomalies.

17 Compare the calibre of the veins and arteries.
 ● The normal ratio is 4:3 and in older individuals 3:2.

18 Follow the vessels to the fundus.

19 Note in particular the color and any signs of edema.

20 Next examine the macula (with the patient looking straight into the ophthalmoscope) (Figures 3 and 5).

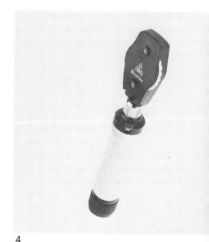

4

21 Here, too, note color, pigment deposits, and any signs of hemorrhage.

22 Examine the retina carefully too.

23 Note hemorrhages, color changes, retinal detachment, tumors or swellings and signs of inflammation.
 ● Exudates have a great diagnostic importance.

24 Record your findings.

25 Compare right and left.

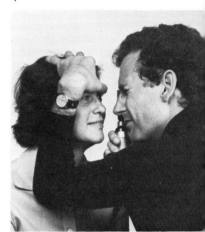

5

26 After completion of the examination, and certainly in patients older than 40 years, administer a few drops of 2% pilocarpine to neutralize the dilation (Figure 6).

27 Remind the patient that he or she will see poorly for a while.

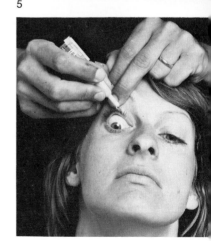

6

Purpose
To obtain an impression of the mobility of the eyes and of the spontaneous movements.

Procedure
1 Ask the patient to look straight ahead.

2 Note whether the eyes stay still or show spontaneous movements (nystagmus).

3 If you find nystagmus, describe:
  - the form,
  - the frequency (rapid or slow),
  - the amplitude (wide or narrow),
  - the direction (of the rapid phase),
  - the degree (first, second or third),
  - the duration (days or weeks).

4 Note whether both eyes look straight forward or one or other deviates.

5 If necessary, make use of a small light source to see whether its reflection on the moist cornea is at the same place in the left and right eye (Figure 1).

6 Note whether the pupils change size when the patient looks in different directions (Figure 2).

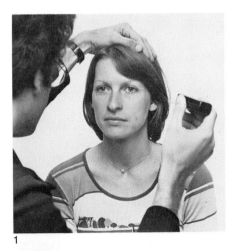

1

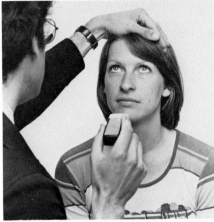

2

D 2.8 Assessment of the eye muscles

Purpose
To obtain an impression of the strength of the eye muscles.

Procedure
1 Assess the strength of the orbicularis muscle of the eye:
   - ask the patient to shut the eyes tight,
   - attempt to push the upper lid up with your thumb (Figure 1),
   - this gives an idea of any difference in strength between the two eyes.
   - If the facial nerve is impaired, the eye on that side cannot be closed. When this condition is present, the eye rolls outward and upward when an attempt is made to close it. (This is known as Bell's phenomenon).

2 Check the extrinsic movements:
   - ask the patient to look straight ahead,
   - to the left,
   - to the right,
   - upward,
   - downward,
   - note any anomalies, restrictions and nystagmus (Figure 2).

3 Check the intrinsic eye muscles (pupil reaction, accommodation reaction).

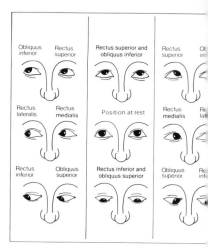

1

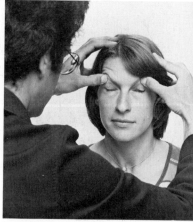

2

2.9 Some eye reflexes

Purpose
To obtain an impression of the neurological efficiency of the eye.

Procedure
1 Examine the corneal reflexes (C 3.3 and Figure 1).

2 Examine the pupil reaction.

3 Examine the accommodation–convergence reflex (Figures 2 and 3):
   - ask the patient to look at a distant object. Now ask the patient to look at your finger as it moves toward the patient's nose.
   - move your finger toward the patient's nose,
   - note the change in the position of the eyes,
   - and in the size of the pupils.

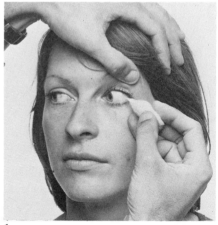

1

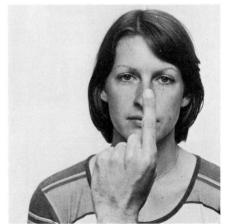

2

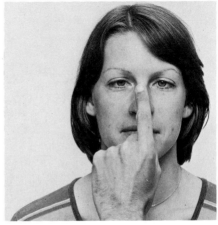

3

D 2.10 Vision and color vision

Purpose
To measure visual acuity, and to obtain an impression of the ability to distinguish colors.

Procedure

A Vision

1 Patients should be asked to wear their glasses for distance correction, but not those for reading.

2 Use Snellen's chart (or some other type) for adults and a picture chart for children (Figures 1 and 2).

3 The patient's chair should be 6 metr from the chart.

4 The chart should be evenly lit with a good light source.

5 Ask the patient to cover the left eye one hand.

6 Test the right eye.

7 Note down the last row of letters tha the patient can still read well.

8 Then test the left eye.

9 Now test both eyes together.

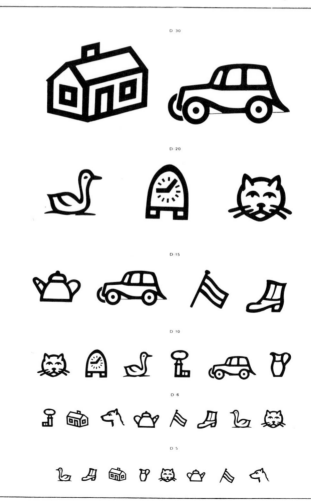

1

B Color vision (using testing color charts)

1 Ask the patient to name the shapes
  seen.
  ● If all the shapes are identified correctly,
  the patient is not color blind

2 When the patient identifies wrong
  shapes, use both combination and
  deduction to determine the anomaly
  from which he suffers.
  ● With the standard tests, any disorder of
  color vision can be detected.

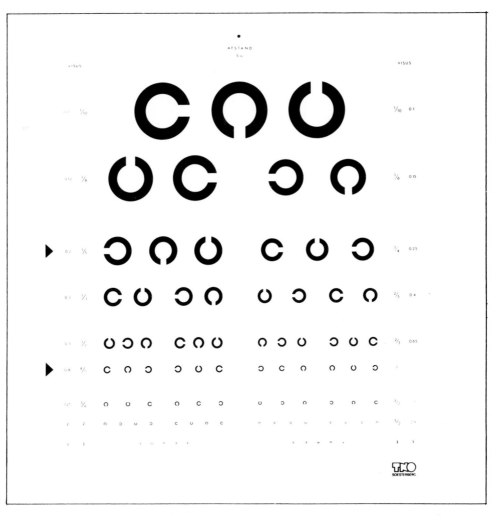

D 2.11 The field of vision

Purpose

To roughly determine the field of vision of the eyes, tested separately.

Procedure

1 Stand in front of the patient.

2 Test the eyes separately by keeping one covered.

3 Ask the patient to look straight ahead and focus on some point (e.g. your nose).

4 Move your finger in a vertical plane, starting high above the patient's line of vision.

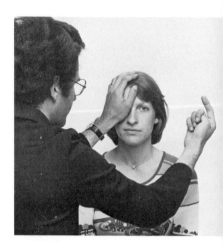

5 Ask the patient to indicate when he sees your finger appear.

6 Record your findings.

7 Then test the other eye.
- This test gives a very rough impression of the field of vision.
- More exact information can be obtained with appropriate instruments.

Purpose
To measure the pressure in the eyeball.

Procedure
• A specialized test that requires the use of a tonometer.

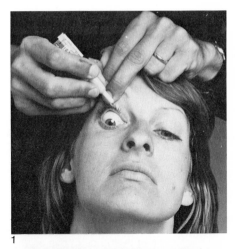

1 Ask the patient to sit down.

2 Administer a local anesthetic agent (e.g. Benoxinate) in the form of eye drops to both eyes (Figure 1).

3 Stain both conjunctivae with fluorescein (D 2.3).

4 Apply the tonometer to the cornea (Figure 2).

5 Look through the tonometer (with the light on) and note what you see.

6 Turn the knob on the tonometer until equilibrium has been reached.
 • The exact procedure is dependent on the type of tonometer used.

7 Read the intra-ocular pressure in mmHg.

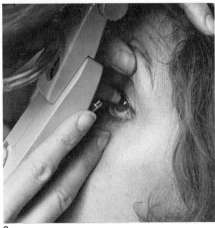

1

2

D 2.13 The lachrymal system

Purpose

To obtain an impression of the patency
of the lachrymal ducts.

Procedure

1 Perform the fluorescein test in each eye
separately (D 2.3).

2 Ask the patient to use a handkerchief
and blow the nose on the side which
has received fluorescein.
- If the handkerchief shows fluorescein
the lachrymal duct on that side is patent.

3 Another way to test patency is to place
an applicator in each nostril and check
for the appearance of dye on the cotton
wool.

3   Examination of the mouth and throat

Purpose
To obtain an impression of the shape, function, and condition of the oral and pharyngeal cavities.

Procedure
1 The patient is seated comfortably in a chair with the head supported at the neck.

2 Ask the patient to open his mouth wide.

3 Have good illumination.

4 Start by examining the teeth, tongue, mucous membranes, the inside of the cheeks, the floor of the mouth and the palate.

5 Then examine the pharynx and the larynx.

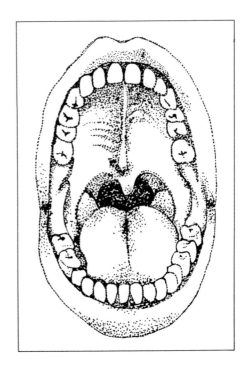

D 3.1 Inspection of the teeth

Purpose
To establish the developmental state of the teeth (quantitatively and qualitatively).

Procedure
1 The patient is seated or supine.

2 Ask the patient to open his mouth wide.

3 Have good illumination.

4 If necessary, use a spatula to push the cheeks and tongue away from the teeth.
   ● Each tooth that has emerged at least halfway is counted.

5 Distinguish between 'milk' and permanent teeth.

6 Make a survey of the teeth present.

7 Evaluate the position of, and distance between, the teeth in the upper and lower jaws.

8 Inspect each tooth separately.

9 Note the size, color, any malformations, plaque, tartar, lesions, or tumors.

10 Pay special attention to the roots of the teeth and the gums (redness and pain).

11 Test each tooth for pain on tapping.

12 Check each tooth for looseness.

13 Note general characteristics such as oral hygiene and the presence of bad breath.

14 Evaluate occlusion of the two jaws.

milk teeth

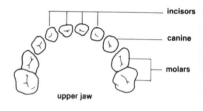

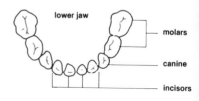

upper jaw

lower jaw

Order of eruption of milk teeth

1. medial lower incisors	6–9 mon
2. medial upper incisors	8–12 mon
3. lateral upper incisors	8–12 mon
4. lateral lower incisors	12–18 mon
5. first molar	12–14 mon
6. canines	end of second ye
7. second molar	first half of third ye

permanent teeth

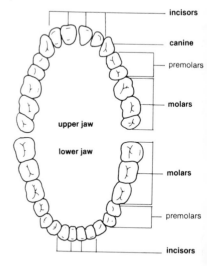

upper jaw

lower jaw

Order of eruption of permanent teeth

1. first true molar	about 6 yea
2. replacement of first incisor	about 7 yea
3. replacement of second incisor	about 8 yea
4. replacement of first molar	about 9 yea
5. replacement of second molar	about 10 yea
6. replacement of incisor	about 11 yea
7. eruption of second molar	about 12 yea
8. eruption of third molar	about 20 yea

Milk or temporary teeth

	Calcification (age in months)		Eruption (age in months)		Transition (age in years)	
	Onset	Completion	Upper jaw	Lower jaw	Upper jaw	Lower jaw
medial incisors	4th fetal	18−24	6−10 (2)	5−8 (1)	7−8	6−7
lateral incisors	5th fetal	18−24	8−12 (4)	7−10 (3)	8−9	7−8
canines	6th fetal	30−39	16−20 (6)	16−20 (6a)	11−12	9−11
first molars	5th fetal	24−30	11−18 (5)	11−18 (5a)	9−11	10−12
second molars	6th fetal	36	20−30 (7)	20−30 (7a)	9−12	11−13

Permanent teeth

	Calcification		Eruption	
	Onset (months)	Completion (years)	Upper jaw (years)	Lower jaw (years)
medial incisors	3−4	9−10	7−8 (3)	6−7 (2)
lateral incisors	upper: 10−12 under: 3−4	10−11	8−9 (5)	7−8 (4)
canines	4−5	12−15	11−12 (11)	9−11 (6)
first premolars	18−24	12−13	10−11 (7)	10−12 (8)
second premolars	24−30	12−14	10−12 (9)	11−13 (10)
first molars	birth	9−10	5½−7 (1)	5½−7 (12)
second molars	30−36	14−16	12−14 (12)	12−13 (12a)
third molars	upper: 7−9 lower: 8−10	18−25	17−30 (13)	17−30 (13a)

Numbers in parentheses indicate the order of eruption. Many otherwise healthy children do not conform exactly with this sequence. (From Silver H.K. *et al.* (1974). *Kindergeneeskunde* (Paediatrics); 2nd ed. (Utrecht).

D 3.2 Percussion of the teeth

Purpose
To obtain an impression of the
condition of the teeth by percussion.

Procedure
1 Ask the patient to open his mouth wide.

2 Have good illumination.

3 Tap each tooth systematically.

4 Tap with a metal rod.

5 Ask the patient to say whether he feels
pain.

6 Compare right, left, upper and lower.

7 Attempt to form an impression of the
patient's pain threshold.

D 3.3 Inspection of the tongue

Purpose
To obtain an impression of the shape
and condition of the tongue by
inspection.

Procedure
1 Ask the patient to open his mouth wide.

2 Inspect the tongue.

3 Note the shape of the tongue in
particular.

4 Note whether the tongue is symmetrical.

5 Note whether fasciculation is present.

6 Ask the patient to stick out the tongue.

7 Note whether the tongue lies straight
out, or deviates to the right or left.

8 Note the color of the tongue, the
presence of any fur and any ulceration

9 Note the moistness of the tongue.

D 3.4 Testing of taste

Purpose
To obtain an impression of the taste
function of the tongue.

Procedure
1 Test the taste sensitivity with:
- sweet: a 20% sugar solution,
- sour: a 10% saline solution,
- acid: a 5% citric acid solution,
- bitter: a 1% quinine solution.

2 Make certain that the patient keeps the
tongue extended until he has determined
the taste.

3 Make certain that the patient's nose is
completely blocked.

4 Test both halves of the tongue.
●The anterior two-thirds of the tongue is
enervated by the chorda tympani, the
posterior one-third by the
glossopharyngeal nerve.

Inspection of the mucous membranes

Purpose

To obtain an impression of the condition of the mucous membranes of the mouth.

Procedure

1 Sit in front of the patient.

2 Ask the patient to open his mouth wide.

3 Have very good illumination (Figure 1).

4 Inspect the mucous membranes of the mouth systematically.

5 Inspect the mucous membranes around the teeth and gums (Figure 2).

6 Inspect the mucous membranes of the walls of the cheeks (Figure 3).

7 Inspect the mucous membranes of the floor of the mouth (Figure 4), having asked the patient to raise and retract the tongue.

8 Inspect the mucous membranes of the posterior wall of the pharynx.

9 While inspecting, pay special attention to color, tumors or swellings, secretion, any inflammation, degree of moistness, ulceration, and petechial hemorrhages.

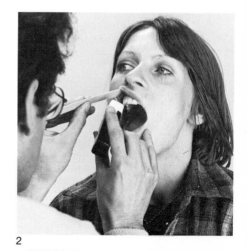

2

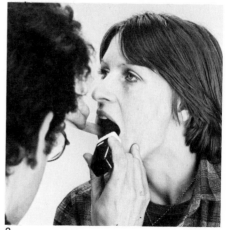

3

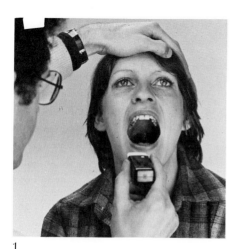

1

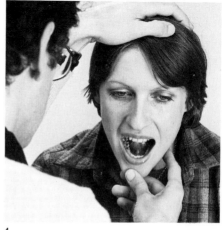

4

D 3.6 Palpation of the cheeks

Purpose
To obtain an impression of the shape
and any anomalies of the cheeks as
well as of the structures in this area.

Procedure
1 Sit in front of the patient.

2 Ask the patient to open his mouth wide.

3 Take hold of the cheek between thumb
and index finger, the former inside the
mouth and the latter outside it (see
Figure 1).

4 Check the cheek systematically.

5 Look in particular for tumors or
swellings.

6 If you find a swelling, attempt to
determine the size, consistency,
relationship with the surroundings, and
painfulness, if any.

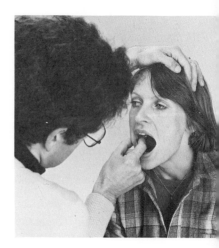

Palpation of the floor of the mouth

Purpose
To obtain an impression of the shape (and any anomalies) of the structures in the floor of the mouth.

Procedure

1 Sit facing the patient.

2 Ask the patient to open the mouth wide.

3 Ask the patient to bend the tongue backward as if saying 'el'.

4 Palpate the floor of the mouth with the index finger of your right hand (see Figure 1).

5 If necessary, apply counterpressure with your thumb under the chin.

6 Look in particular for any swellings.

7 Assess the opening of the submaxillary, sublingual, and submandibular ducts.

8 Check the frenulum of the tongue.

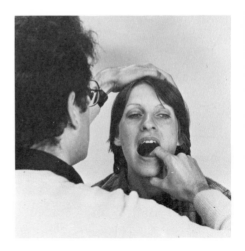

D 3.8 Inspection of the palate

Purpose
To obtain an impression of the roof of the mouth by inspection.

Procedure
1 Under good illumination, inspect both the hard and the soft palate (see Figure 1).

2 Note in particular the shape of the roof of the palate (bony skeleton).

3 Look for swellings and fissures, and check symmetry.

4 Check the symmetry of the soft palate in particular.

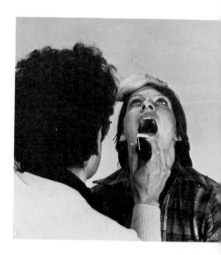

9 Palpation of the palate

Purpose
To obtain an impression of the roof of
the mouth by palpation.

Procedure
1 Ask the patient to open the mouth wide.

2 Palpate the palate with your index
finger, particularly the hard palate.

3 Watch especially for fissures and
swellings.

D 3.10 Inspection of the pharynx

Purpose

To obtain an impression of the shape of
the pharynx and the condition of the
mucous membranes.

Procedure

1 Sit facing the patient.

2 Have very good illumination.

3 Ask the patient to open the mouth.

4 Press the tongue down gently with a
spatula and ask the patient to say 'Ah'
(see Figure 1).

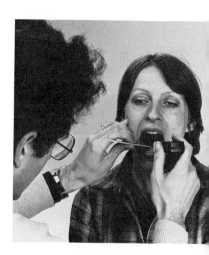

5 This opens the pharynx to its maximum
and you can inspect successively:
- the uvula,
- the tonsils,
- the posterior wall of the pharynx and
the glands.

6 Pay special attention to the mucous
membranes and any signs of
inflammation or pus secretion.

Purpose

To obtain an impression of the shape of the internal and external larynx and the laryngeal structures.

Procedure

A The internal larynx

1 Use can be made of direct and indirect laryngoscopy.
   • The indirect method produces more information.

2 Have a very good light source.

3 The patient's mouth must be wide open.

4 Choose a throat mirror (relatively larger than the one used for posterior rhinoscopy).

5 Warm the mirror to body temperature (check on the back of your hand).

6 Ask the patient to stick out the tongue.

7 Wrap a square of gauze around the tongue to aid in holding it in place (Figure 1).

8 Introduce the mirror, which should be facing downward (Figure 2).

9 Push the uvula gently upward with the mirror.

10 Ask the patient to say 'Ah'.

11 Advance the mirror carefully, touching the posterior wall of the pharynx as little as possible.

12 Turn the mirror to the right and to the left, forward and backward, and tilt it (Figures 3 and 4).

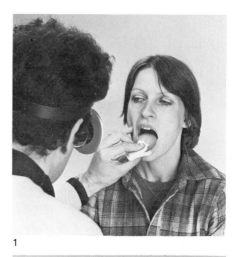

1

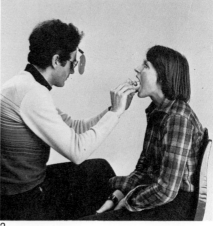

2

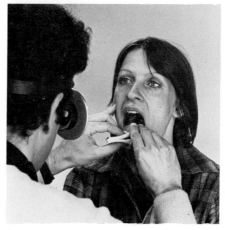

3

13 This makes it possible to inspect the piriform sinus, the anterior and posterior parts of the glottis and the vocal cords.

14 Indirect laryngoscopy gives an impression of, successively:
 - the base of the tongue,
 - the epiglottis,
 - the piriform sinus,
 - a large part of the structure of the larynx,
 - the two vocal cords (mobility),
 - the posterior and anterior parts of the glottis.

15 Look for any deviation in shape and color and for the presence of any secretions.

16 If you do not form a clear impression of the larynx, you will have to arrange to have direct laryngoscopy performed.

B The external larynx

1 Sit straight in front of the patient.

2 Under good illumination, examine the shape and course of the larynx.

3 Look in particular for any swellings.
 •Thyroid gland tissue follows the movements of swallowing.

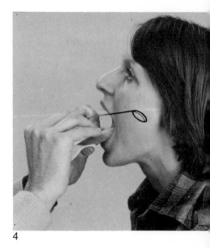

4

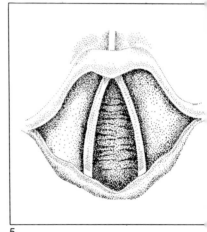

5

3.12 Palpation of the larynx

Purpose
To obtain an impression of the shape
and course of the larynx by inspection.

Procedure

1 Sit or stand in front of the patient.

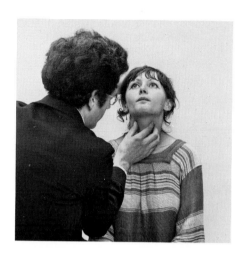

2 Place your thumb on one side of the
larynx and your other fingers on the
other side (see Figure 1).

3 Palpate systematically downward.

4 Palpate the skin and superficial tissues
first.

5 Palpate the bony elements of the larynx
next (the hyoid bone, and the thyroid
and cricoid cartilage).

6 Attempt to form an impression of the
anatomy of the larynx.

7 Attempt to form an impression of the
course of the larynx.

8 Look in particular for any swellings.
●(Aberrant) thyroid gland tissue moves in
conjunction with swallowing
movements.

D 3.13 Examination of the voice

Purpose
To obtain an impression of the quality of the voice.

Procedure
• Disorders of the vagus nerve are manifested by hoarseness.

1 You can evaluate the movement of the vocal cords (D 3.11) or have this done by a specialist.

2 You can have the voice evaluated by a speech therapist.

Examination of the nose

Purpose
To obtain an impression of the shape
and function of the nose.

Procedure
1 The patient should be seated.

2 Start the examination with the external
  nose.

3 Then examine the internal nose.

4 Palpate the adenoids.

5 Examine the area of the sinuses.

6 Test the sense of smell and the patency
  of the nose.

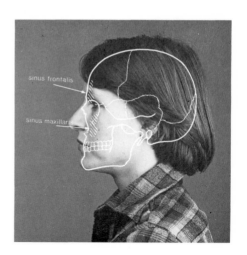

D 4.1   Inspection of the external nose

Purpose
To obtain an impression of the shape of
the nose.

Procedure
1 Sit down facing the patient.

2 Inspect the outside of the nose under
   good lighting.

3 Inspect the nose from the front, from
   the side and from above.

4 Note the shape of the bony part of the
   nose as seen from these angles.

5 Inspect the cartilaginous part of the
   nose.

6 Evaluate the symmetry of the nostrils.

7 Evaluate the skin (color, swellings,
   scars and so on).

8 Lastly, palpate the external nose.

Palpation of the external nose

Purpose
To obtain an impression of the state of
the external nose by palpation.

Procedure

1 Sit down in front of the patient.

2 Palpate the bony part of the patient's
  nose (Figure 1).

3 Palpate the cartilaginous part of the
  patient's nose (Figure 2).

4 Note abnormalities of the skin, bone,
  and cartilage.

5 Assess the mobility of the nasal septum
  by palpation (Figure 3).

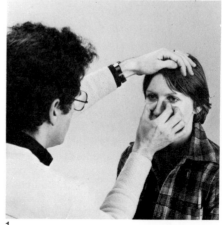

1

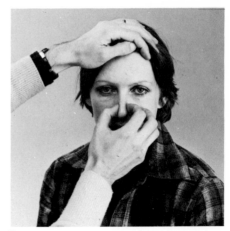

2

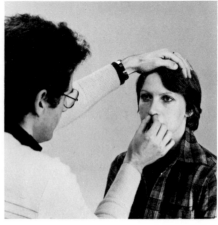

3

D 4.3 Inspection of the internal nose

Purpose
To obtain an impression of the condition of the inside of the nose.

Procedure

A Anterior rhinoscopy

1 Sit down facing the patient.

2 Place the reflecting mirror on your head in the correct position.

3 Switch on a lamp placed behind the patient and shining on the mirror.

4 Adjust the mirror to illuminate the nostril you are about to inspect (Figure 1).

5 Inspect the anterior part of the nostril after elevating the tip of the nose by light pressure with your thumb (Figure 2).

6 Look for septal deviation or subluxation of the septum.

7 Inspect the area of the inferior turbinate.

8 For inspection of the nasal cavity you will need a nasal speculum (Figure 3).

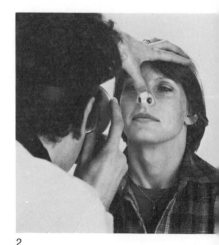

2

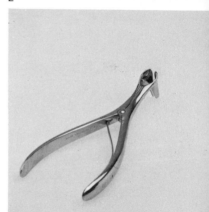

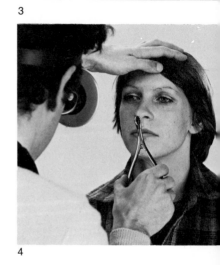

3

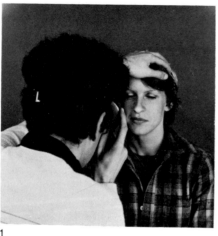

1

9 Place the blades of the speculum in the nasal orifice and spread them (Figure 4).

10 Start by bending the patient's head slightly forward to facilitate inspection of the floor of the nasal cavity (Figures 5 and 6).

11 Then push the head slightly upward to view the upper part of the cavity (Figures 7 and 8).

12 Note the shape and position of the nasal septum.

13 Inspect the nasal isthmus.
   ● This is normally narrow.

14 Inspect the internal cartilages and turbinates.
   ● The lowermost is the most clearly visible.

15 Inspect the nasal mucous membranes (swelling, color and secretion).

16 Lastly, inspect the full nasal cavity, as far as visualization will allow.

17 Remove the speculum carefully, *not* with the blades fully compressed.

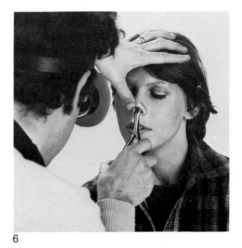

6

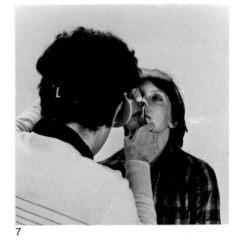

7

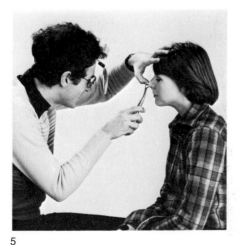

5

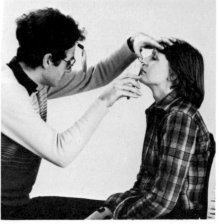

8

B Posterior rhinoscopy

1 Put on the head mirror.

2 Place a light source behind the patient's head and direct it at the mirror.

3 Adjust the mirror to direct the light beam into the patient's mouth.

4 Ask the patient to open the mouth wide.

5 Warm a small throat mirror to body temperature (check on the back of your hand).

6 Place a spatula on the patient's tongue.

7 Ask the patient to say 'Ah'.

8 Introduce the throat mirror into the back of the throat cavity with the mirror facing upward (Figures 9 and 10).

9 Avoid touching the mucous membranes of the pharynx and the uvula as much as possible.

10 Advance the mirror past the posterior margin of the soft palate, making use of the space on the left or right side of the uvula.

11 Ask the patient to breathe through the nose (this relaxes the soft palate and enlarges the entrance to the epipharynx).

12 Next, inspect all the visible parts (shape, colour and secretion; Figure 11).

13 Inspect the epipharynx, with special attention to the opening of the eustachian tubes.

14 In the middle of the upper side of the epipharynx, look for the adenoids (adenoidal tissue is grooved).

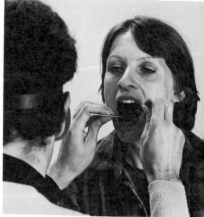

9

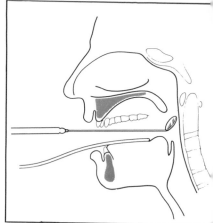

10

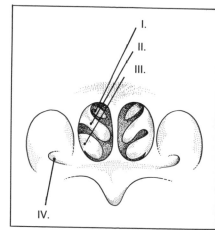

11

4.4 Palpation of the adenoids

Purpose
To estimate the size of the adenoids by palpation.

Procedure

1 Sit facing the patient.

2 Ask the patient to open the mouth wide.

3 Place your index finger in the mouth and follow the soft palate inward.

4 Attempt to go beyond the soft palate with the tip of your finger (see Figure 1).

5 Then flex the distal interphalangeal joint of your index finger.

6 Next, palpate the adenoids in the epipharynx, noting size and any pain.
 • Keep in mind that children seldom undergo this examination with comfort: protect your examining finger by using the other hand to press part of the cheeks between the upper and lower teeth (Figure 1).

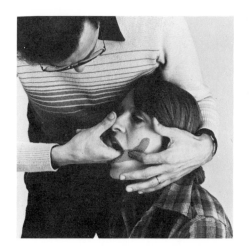

D 4.5 Percussion of the sinuses

Purpose
To obtain, by percussion, the recognition of disease in one or any of the sinuses (Figure 1).

Procedure
1 Sit facing the patient.

2 With your middle finger, tap firmly on the skin above the maxillary and frontal sinuses (Figures 2 and 3).

3 Also percuss the branches of the ophthalmic nerve at the site of the supra-orbital fissure.

4 Then percuss the infra-orbital nerve.

5 At each step, ask the patient to say what is felt.

6 Compare left and right sides.

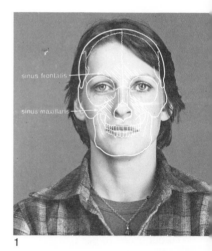

1

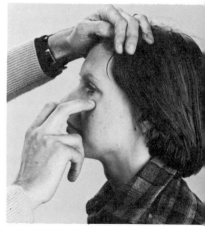

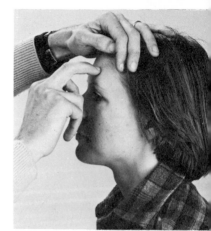

2

3

4.6 Palpation of the sinuses

Purpose
To obtain, by palpation, the recognition of disease in one or any of the sinuses.

Procedure
1 Stand in front of the patient.

2 With both thumbs, press strongly against the skin over the maxillary and frontal sinuses.

3 Press similarly on the branches of the ophthalmic nerve at the site of the supra-orbital fissure (Figure 1).

4 Do the same for the infra-orbital nerve at the site of the infra-orbital foramen (Figure 2).

5 Ask the patient to say what is felt at each step.

6 Compare the left and right sides.

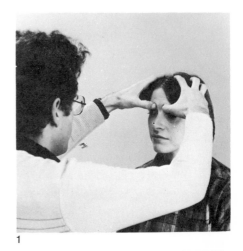

1

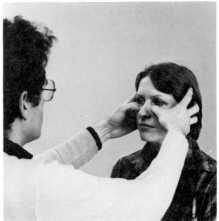

2

D 4.7   Examination of the olfactory sense

Purpose
To obtain an impression of the ability to detect smell.

Procedure
1 The patient is seated with eyes and mouth closed.

2 Test each nostril separately (see Figure 1).
  ● There are special substances to test the sense of smell (coffee powder, nutmeg, pepper).

3 Use these substances if the patient does not smell coffee:
  ● Inability to smell H_2S is an indication of anosmia.
  ● Inability to smell ammonia (function of the trigeminal nerve) indicates that the anosmia is probably psychogenic.

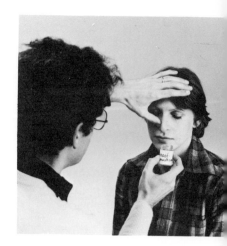

4.8   The patency of the nose

Purpose
To assess any obstruction, defect or
deformity of the lower nasal cavity.

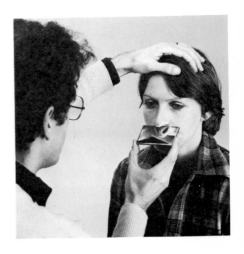

Procedure
1 Sit facing the patient.

2 Use one hand to close one of the
   patient's nostrils and ask the patient to
   blow through the other.

3 Do the same with the other nostril.

4 Note whether the nostril is patent.

5 You can also use a metal mirror for this
   purpose.

6 Place the mirror under the patient's
   nose (see Figure 1).

7 Ask the patient to breathe with the
   mouth closed.

8 Note the area of condensation.

9 Compare the two nostrils.

D 5   Examination of the ears

Purpose
To collect information about the shape
and functioning of the ear.

Procedure
1 Start by examining the external ear up
  to, and including the eardrum.

2 Examine the mastoid process area.

3 Test the hearing.

4 Test the Eustachian tubes.

5 Compare the right and left ears.

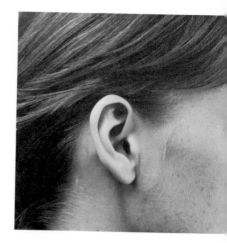

.1 Inspection of the ear

Purpose
To examine the external parts of the ear, including the eardrum.

Procedure
1 The patient should be sitting.

2 You sit facing the patient's side; a child can sit on the lap of the person who has brought him.

3 Use the direct auroscope (Figure 1) for good illumination.
  • Use of a head mirror and a light source is more suitable for treatment procedures, because it leaves both hands free.

4 Start by inspecting the outer ear.

5 Note in particular the shape and position, as well as any abnormalities.

6 Take hold of the top of the ear with your thumb and index finger and draw it backward and upward: this straightens the external meatus and makes the auditory canal visible (Figure 2).

7 Check the entrance to the canal (signs of inflammation, discharge or bleeding etc.).

8 Introduce the tip of the auroscope into the canal (Figure 3).

9 Inspect the wall first.

10 Note the course of the external meatus.

11 Inspect the skin lining the external meatus (scaling, inflammation, injury or wax).

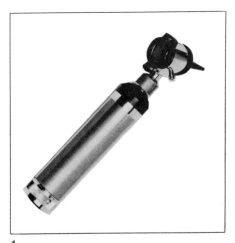
1

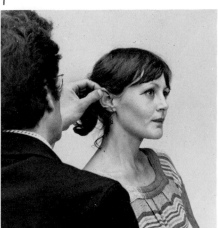
2

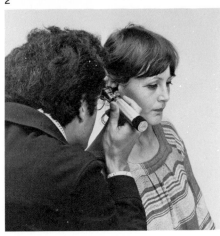
3

12 Then inspect the tympanic membrane
(Figure 4); note the shape, color,
reflectivity, translucency, perforations,
blood, fluid, or evidence of calcification
(anterior or posterior to the eardrum).

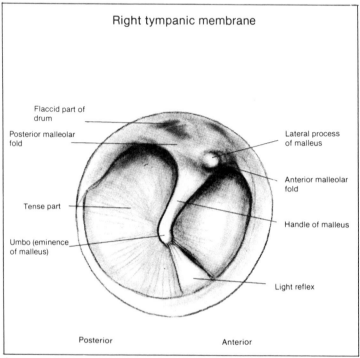

Right tympanic membrane

Flaccid part of drum

Posterior malleolar fold

Lateral process of malleus

Anterior malleolar fold

Tense part

Handle of malleus

Umbo (eminence of malleus)

Light reflex

Posterior

Anterior

4

Palpation of the cartilage and external meatus of the ear

Purpose
To obtain an impression of the state of external ear cartilage by palpation.

Procedure
1 Sit or stand beside the patient.

2 Take hold of the ear with thumb and index finger (Figure 1).

3 Palpate the entire external cartilage systematically.

4 Start with the soft tissues first.

5 Note any pain and swelling.

6 Then palpate the firm part.

7 Note pain, if any.

8 Press the tragus inwards (Figure 2).

9 Press the skull bone under the ear (Figure 3).

10 Note whether this causes pain.
 • Pressure pain at either of these places indicates a disease process in the auditory canal.

11 Compare the left and right sides.

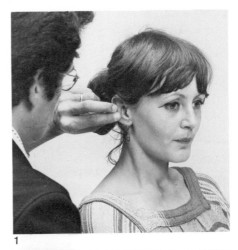
1

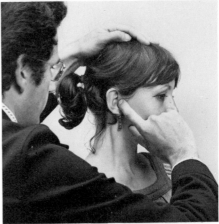
2

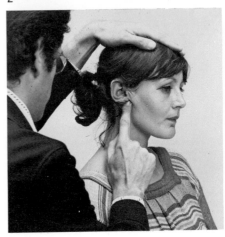
3

D 5.3 Percussion of the mastoid process

Purpose
To obtain an impression of the condition
of the mastoid by percussion.

Procedure
1 Sit or stand next to the patient.

2 With your middle finger bent and using
a wrist action, percuss the mastoid (see
Figure 1).

3 Note whether this causes the patient
pain.

4 Compare left and right.

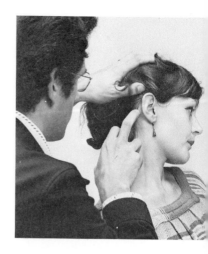

D 5.4 Palpation of the mastoid process

Purpose
To obtain an impression of the mastoid
by palpation.

Procedure
1 Sit or stand next to the patient.

2 Palpate the mastoid with the tips of the
index and middle fingers.

3 Look for swelling and any pain.

4 Compare left and right.

Purpose
To obtain an impression of the patient's ability to hear, or of qualitative and quantitative changes.

Procedure
1 Evaluation of the hearing is a test of function.

2 Hearing is tested after examination of the ear.

3 Start with the whisper test. If the result is good, the hearing function is good; if not, the investigation is continued.

4 The tuning fork examination is performed next.

5 If the results of the tuning fork tests are not satisfactory an audiogram is required.
   • The tone audiogram and speech audiogram must be undertaken by a specialist.

D 5.6 The whisper test

Purpose
To obtain an impression of the quality of the hearing.

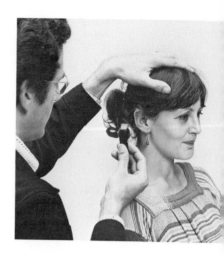

Procedure

1 Ask the patient to stand about 6 meters away with his back to you.

2 Ask him to cover one ear with his hand.

3 Whisper a number (e.g. 66).

4 Ask the patient to repeat what he has heard.

5 Test the other ear in the same way.

6 Compare the left and right ears.

7 You can also use a watch with a quiet tick to obtain an impression of the patient's hearing.

8 Hold the watch against the external ear.

9 Ask whether the patient hears the ticking.

10 Move the watch away slowly (see Figure 1).

11 Ask the patient to say when the ticking of the watch is no longer heard.

12 Compare the right and left ears.

13 Compare with your own hearing.

5.7 The tuning fork examination

Purpose
To evaluate the quality of the hearing with a tuning fork.

Procedure
1 Background noise, in the room where the test is performed, must be reduced as far as possible.

2 Use a tuning fork of 512 Hz.

3 Test one:
   - start the tuning fork vibrating,
   - place its foot on the left mastoid (Figure 1),
   - ask the patient to say when he no longer hears the sound;
   - then hold the tuning fork in front of the patient's left ear, the plane of the fork parallel with that of the external ear (Figure 2),
   - ask the patient whether he still hears the sound of the fork.
   - Normally, air conduction is better than bone conduction (tuning fork beside the ear, versus against the mastoid). Test the other ear in the same way.

4 Test two:
   - start the tuning fork vibrating,
   - place its foot on the middle of the patient's forehead (Figure 3),
   - ask the patient in which ear the tuning fork sounds loudest.

5 Record the results of the tests.

6 Determine whether there is any disturbance of bone or air conduction or a combination of the two.

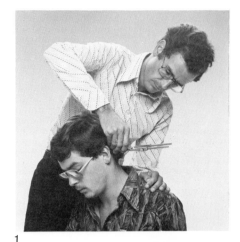

1

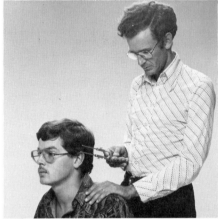

2

	conduction deafness	perception deafness
(1)	negative	positive (normal)
(2)	loudest for affected ear	loudest for unaffected ear

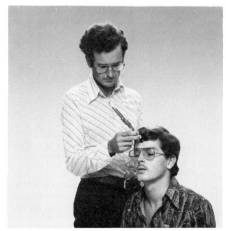

3

D 5.8   Screening audiometry

Purpose
To screen the hearing in each ear separately.

Procedure
1 Use a room with as little background noise as possible.

2 Place the patient with his back to the audiometer.

3 Place the ear-phone of the audiometer over the patient's left ear (Figure 1).

4 Ask the patient to raise his hand when a sound is heard.

5 For each frequency, start testing at 25 dB (lowest intensity). If the patient hears that, further testing at the frequency in question is not necessary.

6 If the patient does not hear 25 dB at a given frequency, perform a systematic examination with the audiometer.

7 For each frequency, record the lowest volume at which the patient still hears a sound. If you are uncertain about the accuracy of your measurements, re-test later (e.g. after testing the other ear).

8 Enter the findings on an audiogram form.

9 Test the other ear.

10 Combine these findings with the results of the tuning fork tests.

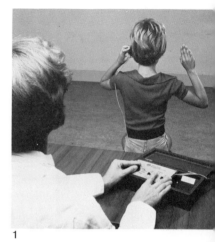

1

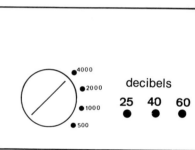

2

5.9   Assessment of the Eustachian tubes

Purpose
To obtain an impression of the
functioning of the Eustachian tubes.

Procedure
1 The patient should be seated.

2 Explain what you are about to do.

3 Ask the patient to close both nostrils
   with the fingers, then to attempt to blow
   the nose, by forced exhalation with the
   mouth firmly closed.

4 The patient may then feel an 'opening of
   the ear'.
   ● The effect of the inflation can also be
   evaluated by auroscope (correction of a
   retracted eardrum).

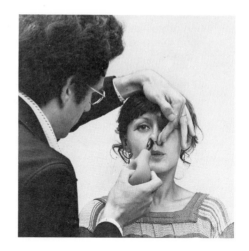

D 6   Examination of the head and neck

Purpose
To obtain an impression of the shape
and function of the neck and the related
organs.

Procedure
1 Ask the patient to undress to the waist.

2 Start the inspection, and include front,
   back and sides.

3 After that, perform auscultation.

4 Next, palpate the neck.

5 Estimate the mobility of the cervical
   spine.

6 Measure the circumference of the neck.

7 Record your findings.

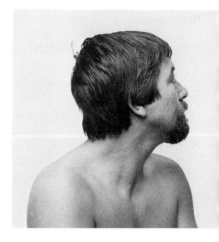

6.1 Inspection of the neck

Purpose
To obtain an impression of the shape of the neck and the structures in it, by inspection.

Procedure

1 Ask the patient to undress to the waist.

2 Have good illumination.

3 Inspect the front, the back and the sides of the patient's neck.

4 Compare the right and left sides.

5 Perform the inspection systematically.

6 Start in the midline of the front of the neck.

7 Note the position of the head at the same time.

8 Note the position and course of the larynx.

9 Look for local swellings:
   - in the supraclavicular area,
   - in the lateral cervical triangle,
   - in the medial cervical triangle,
   - in the suprasternal fossa.

10 Look for pulsating swellings.

11 Look for dermatological changes (color, atrophy, lesions, swellings, scars and hair).

D 6.2 Palpation of the cervical vertebrae

Purpose
To obtain an impression of the shape and mobility of the cervical portion of the spinal column.

Procedure ˙

1 Ask the patient to expose the neck.

2 Stand behind the patient.

3 Palpate the contours of the neck.

4 Look for swellings, inflammation, and any involuntary tension of the muscles.

5 Note any pressure pain.

6 Next, palpate the spinous processes systematically.

7 Percuss the neck vertebrae and note whether the patient feels pain (see Figure).

8 Lastly, perform function tests (D 6.9).

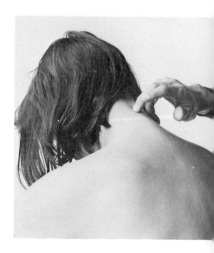

Purpose
To obtain an impression of the presence and location of the lymph glands in the neck.

Procedure
1 Stand in front of the patient.

2 Include the back of the neck in the examination.

3 Palpate the neck systematically (see Figure). In particular check:
   - the occipital glands,
   - the gland along the short neck muscles,
   - the retro-auricular glands,
   - the pre-auricular glands,
   - the submandibular glands.

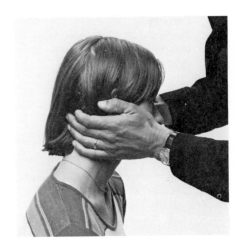

4 For each gland found, determine:
   - the location,
   - the margins,
   - the relationship with the surroundings (skin, deep tissues and other glands),
   - the size,
   - the shape,
   - the consistency,
   - any tenderness.

D 6.4 Palpation of the common carotid artery

Purpose
To obtain an impression by palpation, of the course and any changes in the common carotid artery.

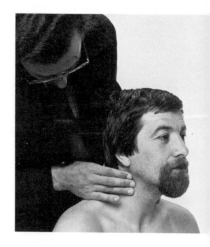

Procedure
1 The patient's neck is exposed.

2 Find the common carotid artery (see Figure).

3 Assess the condition of the vessel walls (thickening, contractions or hardness).

4 Note any palpable thrill or pulsation.

5 Evaluate the rhythm and regularity of the beat.

6 Compare the right and left sides.
  ● Do not palpate the arteries on both sides at the same time; carotid pressure can cause a loss of consciousness (and even cardiac arrest).

Purpose
To obtain an impression by palpation, of the location, size, and consistency of the thyroid gland.

Procedure

1 The patient's neck is exposed.

2 Palpate the suprasternal fossa with your index and middle fingers (Figure 1).

3 Ask the patient to swallow.
   - This makes enlarged glands more easily palpable.
   - Swallowing can be facilitated by giving the patient a sip of water.

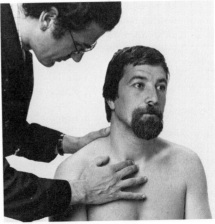

1

4 You can also stand behind the patient and place both hands around his neck, palpating the thyroid gland region with the second and third fingers. Palpation can be performed more accurately if the trachea is held in place on one side (Figure 2).

5 If you feel thyroid gland tissue, determine:
   - the exact extent,
   - the shape,
   - the size,
   - the consistency,
   - and the nature of the surface of the gland.

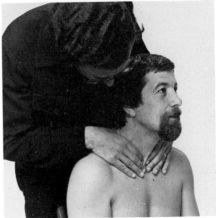

2

6 During palpation, note any vibration or pulsations in the gland.
   - Aberrant thyroid gland tissue moves together with swallowing movements.

D 6.6 Measurement of the circumference of the neck

Purpose
To determine the circumference of the neck as a measure of the growth of any tissues, e.g. goiter.

Procedure
1 The patient's neck is exposed.

2 Circle the patient's neck with a tapemeasure, using the 7th cervical vertebra and the space under the thyroid cartilage as reference points (see Figure).

3 Measure to an accuracy of 0.5 cm.
   •The neck circumference is an individual parameter, and therefore only changes in that individual's measurement have diagnostic value.

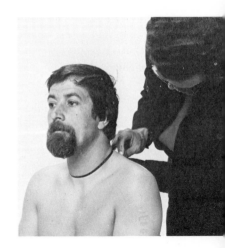

Purpose
To use auscultation to collect information about a possible stenosis of the common carotid artery.

Procedure
1 The patient's neck is exposed.

2 Determine the position of the common carotid artery on both sides.

3 With your stethoscope, listen to the pulsations over the course of the common carotid artery; ask the patient to hold his breath (see Figure).

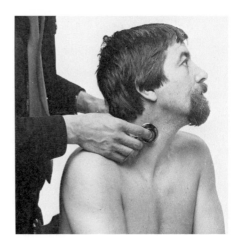

4 Listen for any murmurs.

5 Determine the area of maximum intensity of any murmur.
  ● In the supraclavicular fossa you can hear other vessel sounds as well. These sounds are often conducted heart sounds.

D 6.8   Auscultation of the thyroid gland

Purpose
To collect information about the
vascularity of the thyroid gland by
auscultation.

Procedure

1 The patient's neck is exposed.

2 Place your stethoscope on the larynx,
   just above the upper edge of the
   sternum (see Figure).

3 Try to detect any vascular sounds that
   might indicate the presence of a goiter,
   or other disorders.

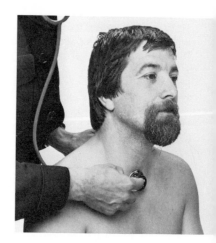

Evaluation of the functioning of the cervical portion of the spinal column

Purpose
To assess the mobility of the cervical part of the spinal column.

Procedure
1 The patient's neck and upper trunk are exposed.

2 Stand at the back of the patient.

3 Test the active mobility by asking the patient to perform the following movements:
   - anteflexion,
   - dorsiflexion,
   - lateral flexion to the right and the left,
   - rotation to the right and left.

4 Determine the degree of mobility.

5 Test the same movements passively (Figures 1–6).

6 For this purpose, take the patient's head between your hands and perform the same movements as done under 3.

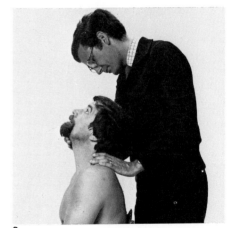

1

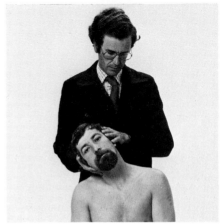

2

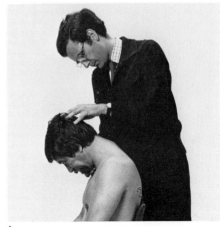

3

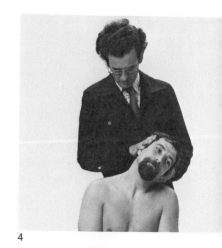

4

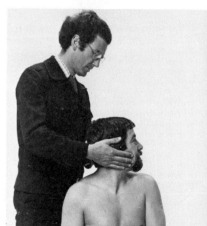

5

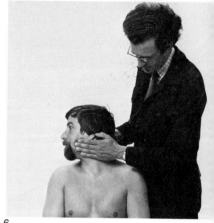

6

7 Examination of the thorax

Purpose
To obtain an impression of the shape and function of the thorax and the internal organs in this region by inspection, palpation, percussion and auscultation.

Procedure
1 The patient's body is exposed to the waist.

2 The patient's position is dependent on the phase of the examination and his condition, e.g. it may be performed with the patient sitting or standing.

3 Make certain that your hands, the room and the stethoscope are warm.

4 Explain to the patient what you are about to do.

5 Remember to examine four sides: front, back, right and left.

6 Start by inspecting the thorax.

7 In recording your findings, always indicate the site: in front, for instance, in relation to the ribs (horizontal) and the thorax (vertical), and on the back in relation to the spinous processes starting with the 7th cervical vertebra and (when orientation is difficult) relative to the point of the scapula (at the level of the 8th thoracic process) as horizontal orientation points, and the scapular line and the paravertebral lines as vertical orientation points (Figures 1 and 2).

8 Next, assess the respiration and the lungs.

9 Then proceed with the heart.

10 It may be necessary to have further tests done, e.g. to determine the central venous pressure, the blood pressure and to obtain an ECG.

11 It will often suffice to examine only part of the thorax (e.g. only the lungs or the breasts).

12 Ask the patient to dress; do not leave the patient unclothed longer than is necessary for the examination.

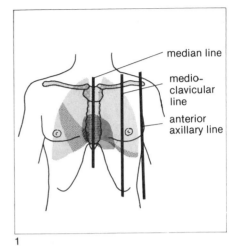

median line
medio-clavicular line
anterior axillary line

1

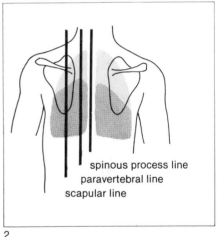

spinous process line
paravertebral line
scapular line

2

D 7.1   Inspection of the skin of the thorax

Purpose
To obtain an impression, by inspection, of the skin of the thorax.

Procedure
1 Inspect according to general principles (A 1).

2 Check in particular the configuration of the thorax (ribs, sternum and spinal column).

3 Note any deviation in shape.

4 Look for any pulsations (intercostally and at the base of the heart).

5 Look for intracostal retraction during respiration.

6 Note any scars (from fistulas, thoracotomy and the like).

7 Look for any evidence of venous congestion or excessive prominence.

7.2 Inspection of the shape of the thorax

Purpose

To obtain an impression, by inspection, of the shape of the thorax and any abnormalities.

Procedure

A General inspection

1 Compare the right and left sides.

2 Inspect the front, sides and back.

3 Inspect at rest, during inspiration and during exhalation.

4 The patient should be relaxed, whether standing, sitting or lying down. The right and left arms should be in the same position (Figure 1).

B The front

5 Inspect the clavicles.

6 Inspect the supra- and infraclavicular fossa.

7 Inspect the sternum.

8 Locate the second rib on both sides.
  • Keep in mind that the ribs do not run horizontally.

9 Note abnormalities in the course or number of the ribs.

C The back (Figure 2)

10 Locate the prominent seventh cervical vertebra.
  • The point of the scapula lies at the level of the eighth thoracic vertebra.

11 Note the course and shape of the vertebral column (e.g. kyphosis or scoliosis).

12 Note the shape and the position that the scapulae are held in.

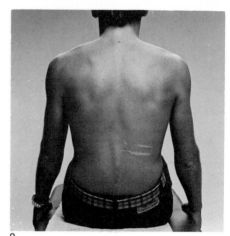

1

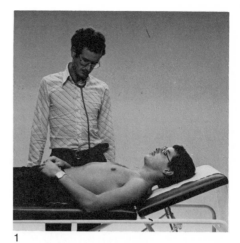

2

D The thoracic skeleton

13 Note the shape of the thoracic skeleton as a whole, e.g. depressed over the sternum, or 'barrel' chested (Figures 3–5).

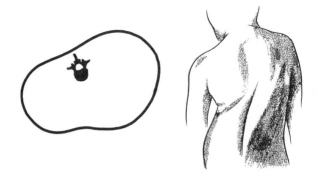

3 Thoracic kyphoscoliosis

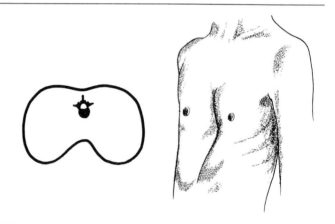

4 Depression of the sternum

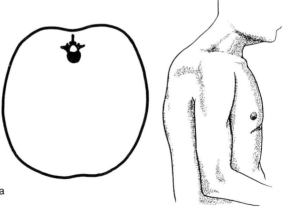

5 The 'barrel' chest, e.g. emphysema

Palpation of the thorax

Purpose
To obtain an impression of the
movements of the thorax by palpation.

Procedure

1 Place both hands flat on the front of the
thorax (Figure 1).

2 Ask the patient to exhale.

3 Palpate the thorax movements.

4 Compare the right and left sides.

5 Standing at the back of the patient,
place your hands on the sides of the
chest (Figure 2).

6 Note the sideward movement of your
hands.

7 Place both hands on the patient's back
(Figure 3).

8 Here too, compare the thoracic
excursion on both sides. The back will
move least, the sides and the front the
most.

9 Vocal fremitus can be detected by
palpation.

10 Ask a patient to use a deep voice and to
say "99".

11 Put your hand on the back of the thorax
while this is done.

12 Compare the vibrations you feel in your
two hands.

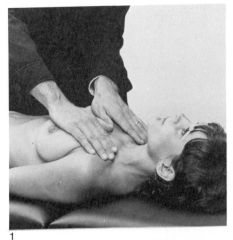
1

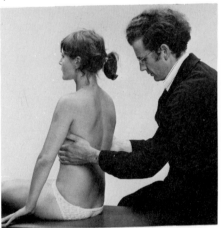
2

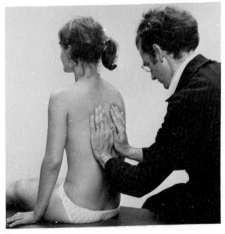
3

D 7.4 Measurement of the circumference of the thorax

Purpose
To obtain quantitative information about the range of the thoracic movements.

Procedure

1 Ask the patient to sit down.

2 Use a flexible tapemeasure placed at the nipple level around the chest (see Figure).

3 Measure the chest circumference at maximal inspiration.

4 Measure the chest circumference at maximal expiration.

5 Record both to an accuracy of 0.5 cm.
  ●The difference between these values should be recorded.

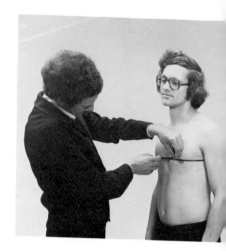

7.5 Percussion of the lungs

Purpose
To use percussion (indirect unless otherwise indicated) of the thorax to obtain information about the boundaries and quality of the tissues so contained.

Procedure

A Anterior (the patient is supine)

1 Compare the right and left sides throughout.

2 Systematically percuss downward (Figures 1 and 2; the position of the heart is obvious with comparative percussion).

3 Percuss the supraclavicular fossa as well (if necessary for a deep-lying fossa, use a curved middle finger to tap the skin, i.e. direct percussion).

4 Also percuss the clavicle (by direct percussion).

5 Next, percuss both sides (ask the patient to raise the arms). Start in the armpit.

6 Locate the margins of the liver (D 7.8).

B Posterior (the patient sitting or standing)

7 Make certain the patient is sitting straight.

8 Start at the top of the lungs (Figure 3).

9 Compare left and right.

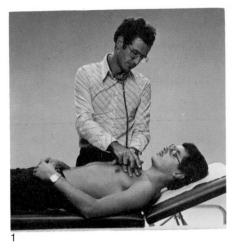

1

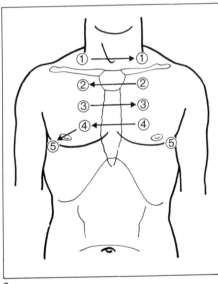

2

10 Percuss downward until the percussion
   tone found over the lungs has entirely
   disappeared.
   •There may be a difference of one
    finger's breadth between the lower
    margin of the right and left lungs (the
    right often being higher because of the
    presence of the liver).
   •Posteriorly, the lower margin is usually
    found at the level of the 10th or 11th
    thoracic spinous process.

11 Determine the respiratory mobility
   (D 7.7).

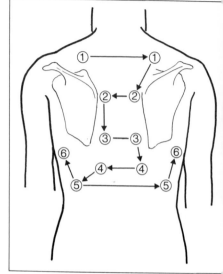

3

Purpose
To establish the presence or absence of changes in the respiratory tract or lungs by means of auscultation.

Procedure
● Auscultation is performed after inspection and percussion.

1 Ask the patient to exhale quietly with an open mouth.

2 Auscultate the thorax systematically (Figures 1 and 2).

3 Listen to one complete inspiration and expiration period each time.

4 Compare right and left.

5 Begin in front above the clavicle.

6 After listening to this area, auscultate the sides of the chest wall.

7 Lastly, auscultate the back of the thorax from top to bottom and comparing right and left at each level (Figure 3).
   ● Normally, you will hear vesicular respiration:
   - soft sounds on inspiration, still softer on expiration.
   - the sounds on inspiration last longer than those on expiration.
   ● Vesicular breathing is usually of equal intensity on both sides, but is sometimes slightly sharper on the right side.

8 Note changes in sound: weaker, sharper, prolonged, sighing, bronchial noises and so on.

9 Check for other sounds (bronchitic, dry rhonchi, moist rhonchi, friction etc.).

10 Indicate the exact place where you have heard abnormal sounds.

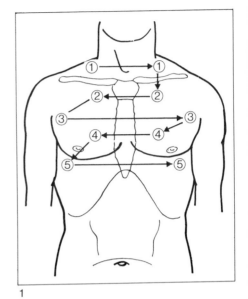

1

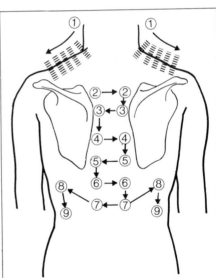

2

11 Determine whether the voice conduction
   is normal:
   - ask the patient to say "66" and compare
     the corresponding right and left lung
     areas.
   ● Normally, this can hardly be heard with
     the stethoscope; strong conduction
     (bronchophony) indicates a pathological
     process.

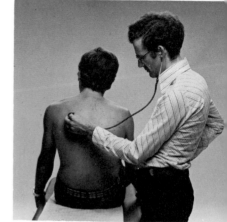

3

Purpose
To establish the movement of the lung boundaries by percussion, to detect the degree of pleural movement or lung elasticity.

Procedure
• The respiratory movements can best be evaluated on the patient's back.

1 Percuss the back from top to bottom.

2 Continue until you reach a place where the sonorous percussion tone disappears.

3 Hold your middle finger on that place.

4 Ask the patient to inhale deeply.

5 Percuss again. You will notice that the dull percussion tone changes into a sonorous tone (in a healthy patient).

6 If the patient holds his breath, percussion further downward will yield a sonorous percussion tone (Figure 1).

7 The difference between the two boundaries is a measure of the respiratory movement and expansion of the lung (Figure 2).

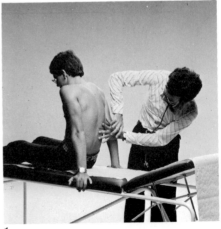

1

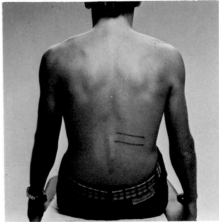

2

D 7.8 Determination of the boundary between the lungs and the liver

Purpose

To determine the lung boundary on the liver side, by percussion.

Procedure

1 Ask the patient to disrobe.
- Percussion on the anterior side of the right lung (see D 7.6) shows a region where the character of the percussion tone changes slightly (becomes shorter).

2 At the level where the liver–lung boundary is expected, percussion must be done very lightly.
- Hard percussion yields the upper margin of the liver and not the lower margin of the lung tissue.

3 Percuss gently in a downward direction (Figures 1 and 2) until the sonorous tone has completely disappeared, after which a dull percussion tone is heard.

4 Indicate this boundary on the skin with a marker pen.
- Normally, this boundary lies between the 5th and 6th ribs.

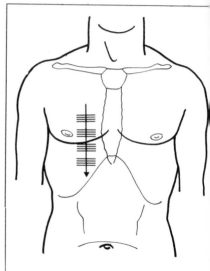
1

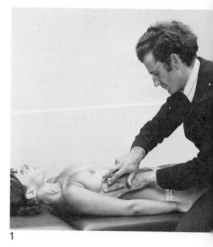
2

Purpose

To inspect the thorax with respect to:
- the influence of the shape on heart and lung function and vice versa, and
- the influence of cardiac anomalies on local movements.

Procedure

1 Make certain that the seated patient's arms are in similar positions, and inspect all four sides.

2 Note any abnormal shape of the skeleton.

3 Look for any precordial bulging of the thorax.

4 Locate and determine the area of the apex beat of the heart.

5 Look for other pulsating swellings, with special attention to the 2nd intercostal space on the left and right sides, the 3rd–5th parasternal intercostal spaces on the left, and in the epigastric region.

6 Note any systolic retraction, especially in the area of the 2nd and 3rd intercostal spaces on the left and right sides.

7 Inspect the skin of the thorax (e.g. for swollen or congested veins etc.).

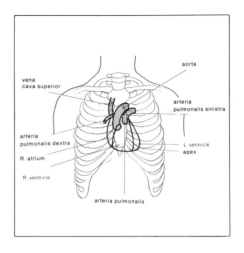

D 7.10 Palpation of the heart region

Purpose
To detect normal and abnormal pulsations in the heart region.

Procedure
1 Palpate with the fingers together — i.e. the flat palmar surface of the hand.

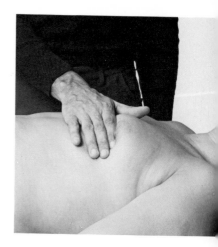

2 Palpate the left side first: lay your hand over the 4th or 5th intercostal space, the fingers a little beyond the medioclavicular line (see Figure).
 - The normal apex beat of the heart is often palpable and very precisely located (it can be felt with one finger).
 - When the heart is enlarged, the apex beat is displaced downward and to the left.

3 Determine not only the site but also the character of the apex beat or the heart, the patient lying on his left side.
 - The sensation felt can be fast and strong, thrusting or vibrating.

4 In the same way, palpate the right side of the heart (2nd or 3rd to 4th or 5th left intercostal space parasternally).

5 Also assess any other vibrations ("thrills") in the heart region.

6 After this palpation, perform percussion.

7.11 Percussion of the heart region

Purpose
To obtain an impression of the position and size of the heart, by percussion.

Procedure
1 The patient is examined in the semi-supine position.

2 Percuss somewhat more forcefully than for the lung—liver boundary.

3 Locate the left margin of the heart first: percuss from the side to the midline under the nipple (see Figure).
 • The percussion tone changes distinctly at the lateral margin (normally just within the medioclavicular line).

4 Next, locate the right margin: percuss above the lung—liver boundary from the side to the midline until the character of the tone changes distinctly.
 • The normal right margin lies at the middle of the sternum.

5 Percuss the upper margin of the heart, normally found in the 3rd intercostal space.
 • These three margins indicate the relative area of the cardiac space, form a measure of the size of the heart, and give an impression of its position.

6 For a more exact determination of the position and size, combine the percussion findings with those obtained by inspection and palpation. X-rays (antero-posterior and lateral, if necessary supplemented with a contrast medium X-ray of the oesophagus) determine the precise area.

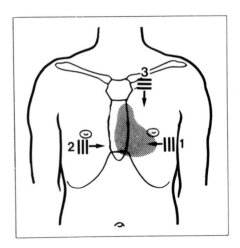

D 7.12 Auscultation of the heart region

Purpose

To obtain an impression of the heart sounds (rhythm and any defects in their character, e.g. murmurs) by auscultation of the heart region.

Procedure

1 By preference, the patient is in a semi-reclining position (about 30°).

2 The examining room must be quiet and peaceful.

3 It must also be warm; otherwise, there may be some shivering or tremor of the thoracic muscles.

4 The patient should breathe steadily in a relaxed way.

5 Concentrate first on the heart sounds and then on any added murmurs.

6 Listen to the *heart sounds* in various places:
   - at the site of the apex beat (with the cup of the stethoscope),
   - in the 2nd intercostal space on the left next to the sternum (with the membrane),
   - in the 2nd intercostal space on the right (with the membrane),
   - in the 4th and 5th intercostal spaces on the left next to the sternum (with the cup).

7 Since the apex beat differs between individuals, care must be taken to locate it accurately.

8 Note the frequency and rhythm of the heart sounds.

9 Distinguish between the systolic and diastolic beats.

10 Attempt to obtain an impression of the intensity of the heart sounds (stronger or weaker than normal, equal or unequal sounds).

11 Note any splitting of sounds, extra sounds, and where they occur in the heart cycle of systole and diastole.

12 Combine this auscultation with a determination of the quality of the pulse at each step.

13 Then determine whether there are systolic or diastolic murmurs.

14 Use both the cup and membrane sides of your stethoscope for this purpose.

15 If no murmurs are heard in the semireclining position, perform auscultation with the patient lying on his side, bending over, and after effort (ten deep knee bends), to find out whether this makes any murmurs detectable.

16 Determine where the murmur is loudest on the chest wall.

17 Determine the direction in which the sound is conducted.

18 Estimate the loudness of the murmur (graded from 1 to 6).

19 Determine when the murmur occurs (pre-systolic, mid-systolic, late systolic, or throughout systole; early diastolic, mid-diastolic, post-diastolic, or throughout diastole).

20 Determine the timbre or character of the murmur (coarse, sibilant, blowing, vibrating, puffing, etc.).

D 7.13 Central venous pressure

Purpose

To determine the central venous pressure as a measure of the mean pressure in the right atrium.

Procedure

1 The patient should be horizontal; it is often necessary to remove the pillow or to place a small pillow under the shoulders.

2 He should breathe normally and be relaxed.

3 Find the place in the neck corresponding with a level 5 cm under the site of attachment of the 2nd rib to the sternum (Figure 1).

4 Observe the venous pulsations in the external jugular vein.

5 If venous pulsations are not visible, ask the patient to press the nostrils closed and to hold the breath.

6 Determine the place where the jugular vein disappears beneath the neck muscles (at this spot the pressure is nil):
- after compression of the cranial end of the vein, or
- after exhalation after the test as in 5 (Figure 2).

7 Determine the difference in level between the spot determined under 6 and where the second rib meets the sternum.

8 This value multiplied by 5 cm gives the central venous pressure.
 •Normally, the venous pressure lies between −3.5 and 1.5.

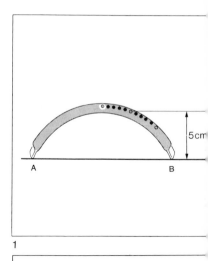

5cm

A   B

1

place where the jugular vein disappears under the neck muscles

jugular vein

2

Purpose
To obtain information about the circulation time of the peripheral circulation.

Procedure

1 Make certain the room is warm; cold surroundings lead to vasoconstriction.

2 Fill a 5 ml syringe with a 20%, or a 10 ml syringe with a 10%, magnesium sulphate solution.

3 Use a large bore needle for the injection.

4 Instruct the patient to indicate if he feels a sensation of warmth in the throat, and to give a second sign when this sensation has disappeared.

5 The patient should be lying down comfortably.

6 Place the arm you are about to inject in full abduction slightly above the level of the thorax.

7 Perform venipuncture of the largest vein in the ante-cubital fossa.

8 Insert the needle well into the blood vessel.

9 Release the tourniquet.

10 Hold the needle firmly in place and inject rapidly with a single stroke, 2.5 ml of the 20% solution, or 5 ml of the 10% solution.

11 Start the stopwatch as you start to inject.

12 Leave the needle in the vein.

13 Read the time between the start of the injection and the moment when the patient gives the pre-arranged sign (appearance and disappearance times).

14 When the sensations have disappeared, repeat the test as a check.

15 Remove the needle, press a pad of cotton wool firmly on the site of injection and hold (or have the patient hold it) until all local bleeding ceases.

16 Have the patient drink some water.
- The normal circulation time is ≥ 15 and ≤ 30 seconds (appearance and disappearance times, respectively).
- The reliability of the test is dependent on the patient's capacity to perceive the described sensation and to react to its presence.
- The reliability of the test is also influenced by the patient's intelligence and willingness to co-operate.

Purpose

To obtain information about heart function by electrocardiography.

Procedure

1 The patient should lie unclothed to the waist and relaxed, on a bed or an examination couch (Figure 2); the temperature of the room must be comfortable.

2 Apply the special contact jelly to the inner side of both wrists and ankles (jewelry etc., must be removed; Figures 3 and 4).

3 Place the electrodes at these sites and close the straps around the wrists and ankles (Figure 5).

4 Attach the four leads to the four electrodes (Figure 6) as follows (where colour-coded):
   - the red lead to the right wrist,
   - the yellow lead to the left wrist,
   - the black lead to the right ankle,
   - the green lead to the left ankle.

5 For the chest (V) there is a fifth (white) lead, which is connected to an electrode attached to the chest in the same way. The sites of these electrodes are as follows (Figures 6 and 7):

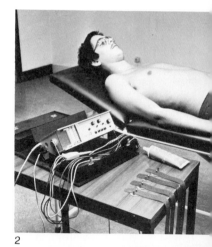

2

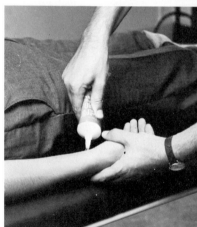

3

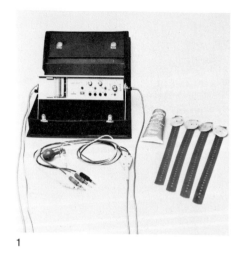

1

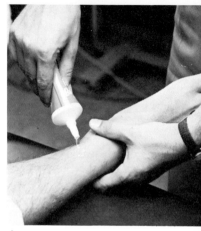

4

- for the V1 lead in the 4th intercostal space on the right edge of the sternum,
- for the V2 in the 4th intercostal space on the left edge of the sternum,
- V3 midway between V2 and V4,
- V4 on the 5th intercostal space on the left medioclavicular line,
- V5 on the anterior axillary line at the level of V4,
- V6 on the mid-axillary line at the level of V4.

6 Prepare the electrocardiograph for use:
- plug in or check that the batteries are demonstrating a sufficient charge,
- attach the patient leads,
- calibrate the instrument by bringing the pen-point to roughly the middle of the paper and the needle's range to 1 cm (= 1 mV).

7 Set the paper speed for 25 or 50 mm/sec, depending on the heart beat rate.

8 Set the lead knob successively at I, II, III, aVR, aVL, aVF, and lastly at V to record the V1−V6 leads, respectively (Figure 8).

9 Register each lead for about 3 seconds.

10 Turn off the electrocardiograph, remove the electrodes, and wipe the jelly off the patient's skin.

11 Put the patient's name and date of birth on the tracing as well as the date of the examination (Figure 9).

12 Note the lead numbers on the tracing.

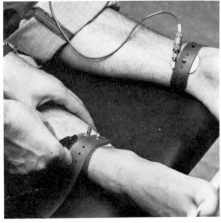

5

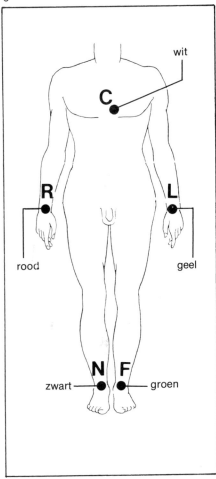

6

155

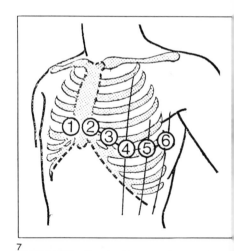

7

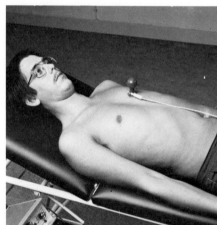

8

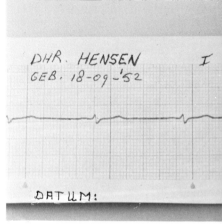

9

7.16 Examination of the breasts

Purpose
To detect any palpable anomalies in the breasts and the regional lymph glands.

Procedure
1 Have the room comfortably warm.

2 Make certain that your hands are warm before palpating.

3 The patient is unclothed to the waist.

A Inspection

4 First inspect while the patient's arms are resting at her sides (Figure 1).

5 Next, inspect while the arms are raised above her head (Figure 2).

6 Then ask her to put her hands on her hips and press (Figure 3).

7 Inspect again after asking her to bend over forwards (Figure 4).

8 Lastly, inspect while she is lying down.

9 While inspecting, note the shape of the breasts.

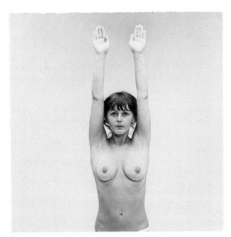

2

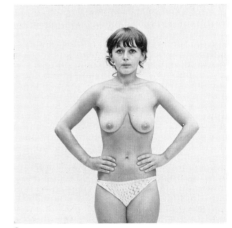

3

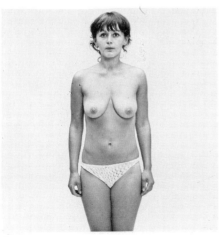

1

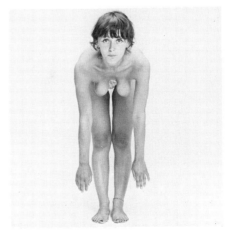

4

10 Assess the symmetry of the breasts and their movements.

11 Inspect the skin for inflammation, atrophy or colour changes.

12 Note any local retractions or protrusions.

13 Pay special attention to the nipples (color, position, shape and evidence of any secretion).

14 Inspect the supraclavicular fossa.

B Palpation

15 Palpate first with your hand flat and the patient standing with her arms resting at her sides (Figure 5).

16 Palpate with the patient's arms raised (Figure 6).

17 Ask her to put her hands on her hips and press before you palpate (Figure 7).

18 Lastly, palpate with the patient lying down. You will collect more information if you put a pillow under the shoulder on the side you are examining (Figure 8).

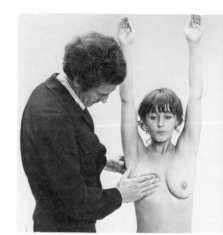

6

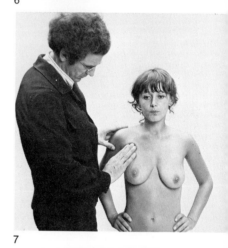

7

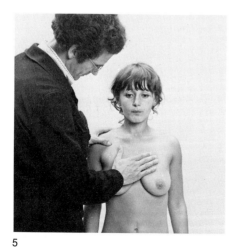

5

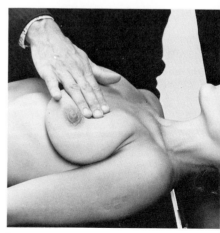

8

19 Palpate the breasts with a flat hand throughout, and make gentle circular movements (Figure 9).

20 Palpate the breasts systematically (center, four quarters and axillary extension).

21 If you feel any firmness of the tissue or resistance to movement, attempt to obtain information about:
- the location,
- the relationship with the skin (attached or not),
- a relationship with the deeper, underlying tissue,
- the shape, and
- the consistency,
- and differentiate from mammary gland tissue.

22 Palpate the supraclavicular fossa (Figure 10).

23 Palpate the armpits (D 7.17).
●Any lumps detected require referral for specialist opinion and if necessary biopsy and histological investigation.

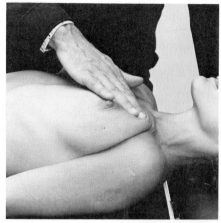

9

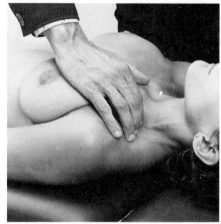

10

D 7.17 Palpation of the axilla

Purpose
To obtain an impression of the anatomy
and any abnormalities of the armpit by
palpation.

Procedure
1 Face the patient.

2 Ask the patient to abduct her arm.

3 Place the closed fingers of your right
   (left) hand in the patient's left (right)
   armpit, your entire hand resting against
   the thorax (Figure 1).

4 Your fingers should point upwards and
   are placed as high as possible.

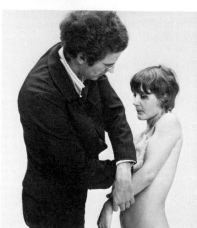

1

5 Ask the patient to move her arm inwards
   towards the chest wall.

6 The arm must rest loose, to avoid
   muscle tension (Figure 2).

7 Palpate from the upper cavity
   downwards with your fingers bent
   slightly at the distal interphalangeal
   joint.

8 Palpate the entire armpit systematically.
   Pay special attention to the upper area
   of the armpit.

9 While palpating, pay special attention to
   any pressure pain and the presence of
   axillary lymph glands.

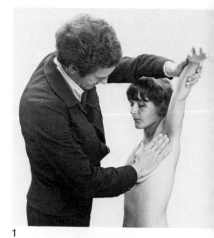

2

10 Determine the shape, size, consistency
    and relationship with the surrounding
    tissues in each case.

Examination of the abdomen

Purpose
To obtain an impression of the shape and functioning of the organs in the abdomen (Figures 1 and 2) by inspection, auscultation, percussion and palpation.

Procedure
1 Ask the patient to undress from the waist down.

2 Have the patient lie down on a firm surface with the head slightly raised on a pillow.

3 Ask the patient to relax; the arms should lie loose alongside the body. If necessary, you can ask him to bend his knees. Ask him to breathe normally. When required, distract his attention by talking to him.

4 Take ample time for the abdominal examination: the interpretation of the findings is very important.

5 Stand or sit on the patient's right.

6 Make certain that the room, your hands and the stethoscope are warm.

7 Tell the patient what you are about to do.

8 Ask him to react to what you do (by describing any pain and other sensations).

9 Start by looking at the patient's abdomen; do not forget the inguinal region.

10 Next, listen to the abdomen with the stethoscope.

11 Then percuss the abdomen.

12 Palpate the abdomen.

13 Examination of the abdomen is almost always followed by a rectal examination.

14 Record the data you have obtained from the examination.

15 Ask the patient to dress.

16 Wash your hands.

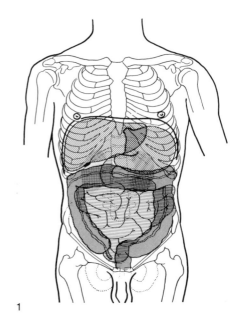

1

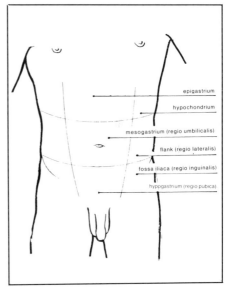

epigastrium

hypochondrium

mesogastrium (regio umbilicalis)

flank (regio lateralis)

fossa iliaca (regio inguinalis)

hypogastrium (regio pubica)

2

D 8.1 Inspection of the abdomen

Purpose
To obtain an impression of the shape of the abdomen and the movements of the abdominal surface.

Procedure
1 Have the patient in the correct position (ref D 8).

2 Note:
   - the general shape of the abdomen,
   - the contours of the abdominal surface,
   - any retractions or protuberances,
   - any asymmetry.

3 Inspect the abdominal skin movement in relation to respiration.

4 Inspect the abdominal skin itself: note hair growth, pigmentation, scars and congested veins.

5 Note the condition of the abdominal muscles.

6 Look for local changes or protrusions (swellings or hernia).

7 Pay special attention to the umbilicus.

8 Inspect the groins; compare left and right, paying special attention to the inguinal folds. Look for swellings, inflammation and pulsations in this region.
   - Inguinal hernias only become visible under elevated abdominal pressure (pressing down, coughing or standing).

9 Continue the examination with auscultation.

8.2 Auscultation of the abdomen

Purpose
To obtain an impression of the functioning of the stomach, intestines, and intra-abdominal blood vessels by auscultation.

Procedure

1 Auscultation is performed after inspection.

2 Place the (warmed) stethoscope just below and to the right of the umbilicus. Press gently and maintain the stethoscope firmly in place (Figure 1).

3 Listening should be prolonged and concentrated.

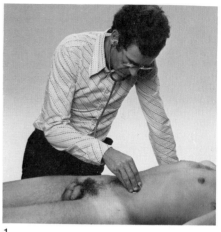

1

4 Next apply the stethoscope in a number of other places, and be sure not to forget the groins (femoral artery, hernial orifices). Work systematically, from upper to lower and from left to right (Figure 2).
  ●You can hear:
   - normal peristalsis,
   - reduced or absent peristalsis,
   - hyper-peristalsis,
   - splashing sounds of fluid present,
   - murmurs and other vascular sounds,
   - friction sounds.

5 Continue the examination with percussion.

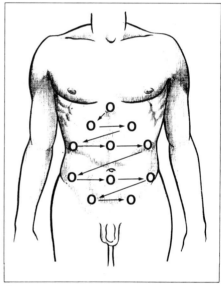

2

D 8.3 Percussion of the abdomen

Purpose

To obtain an impression of the shape and size of the intra-abdominal structures by percussion.

Procedure

1 Percussion is performed after auscultation.

2 Have the patient in the correct position (D 8 and Figure 1).

3 Percuss the entire abdomen systematically (Figure 2).

4 Percuss with the patient lying on the right and left sides (liver and spleen).
- You can detect:
  - high resonance over air space (e.g. gas in the intestines),
  - dull resonance over solid organs (e.g. kidney, spleen etc.).

Pay special attention to:

5 Percussion of the liver and gall bladder area:
  - locate the lung–liver boundary (D 7.8),
  - from there, percuss downward,
  - determine the line between the lower liver border and the abdominal cavity,
  - compare this percussion line with your palpation findings.

6 Percussion of the spleen:
  - the best results are obtained with the patient lying on his right side,
  - percuss the right flank from top to bottom and from front to back.
- When the spleen is enlarged, the dullness of its percussion note will extend further medially and anteriorly and even occupy an area extending to the midline or umbilicus.

7 Percussion of ascites:
  - percuss from the upper boundary of the symphysis pubis upward,
  - determine the boundary of any fluid levels, if present, from the tympanitic sounds of the normal abdomen.

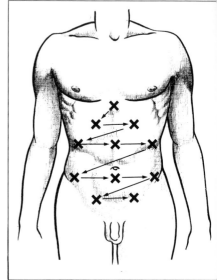

1

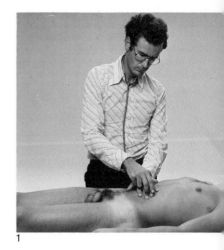

2

- If this line is bordered uppermost by a concave line, ascites is present; if the line has the reverse curve (upward concavity) the bladder is full, the female patient pregnant or a tumor is present.
- Remember that ascites fluid shifts when the patient lies on the side or assumes the knee—chest position; therefore, in these positions other percussion boundaries must be determined.
- Do not attach too much importance to moderate changes in the percussion sounds, especially when not accompanied by other changes (e.g. found on palpation).
- Percussion is particularly useful for the delineation of tumors found at inspection or palpation.

8 Continue the examination with palpation.

D 8.4 Palpation of the abdomen

Purpose
To obtain an impression of the shape, size, and consistency of intra-abdominal organs and structures.

Procedure
● Palpation is performed after inspection, auscultation, and percussion.

1 The patient is appropriately prepared for the examination (D 8).

2 Palpate the entire abdomen systematically.

3 Palpate according to the recommended methods (A 4).

4 Determine any sign of muscular tension or any swelling of the abdomen.

5 Always start at a spot that the patient has indicated as not painful, and proceed slowly towards any indicated painful point.

6 Determine whether pressure pain is felt (pain indicated by the patient on pressure).

7 Determine whether rebound tenderness is felt:
   - press slowly and deeply at a non-painful spot,
   - remove the palpating hand rapidly,
   - ask the patient whether this causes pain at the spot previously indicated.

8 Determine the degree of muscular resistance:
   - press at various places on the abdomen,
   - differentiate between passive and active muscle resistance.

9 Determine the presence of fluid waves:
   - lay the flat hand on one half of the abdomen and the other on the other half,
   - with the first hand, curling the fingers, flick the index finger against the abdominal wall,

   - if you feel a pressure wave with the other hand a few seconds later, fluid may be present.

10 Check for succussion splashing: if present, you can hear it after tapping the abdominal wall sharply with the f of the hand a number of times.

11 Palpate the liver (D 8.5).

12 Palpate the spleen (D 8.6).

13 Then palpate the area of the kidneys, bladder, aorta, iliac artery and determ any areas of discomfort (D 8.7).

Purpose
To obtain an impression of the shape, size, consistency and surface of the liver and the gall bladder by palpation.

Procedure

A The liver

• For optimal palpation, use both hands.

1 Stand to the right of the patient.

2 Place your left hand on the right side of the lumbar region and press forward and upward with slightly bent fingers.

3 Lay your right hand flat on the abdomen under the lowest rib, the fingers pointing obliquely upward, and apply limited pressure (Figures 1 and 2).

4 Ask the patient to inhale deeply.

5 When he does so, you should feel the margin of the liver sliding under the fingers of your right hand.

6 If you feel nothing, palpate higher and/or lower.

7 In many cases you can feel more if during inspiration you press your right hand upward.

8 Locate the margin of the liver, and indicate it as the number of finger-breadths it lies under the lowest rib.
 • If this distance is not more than one finger-breadth, it usually has no pathological significance.

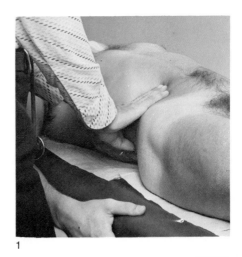

1

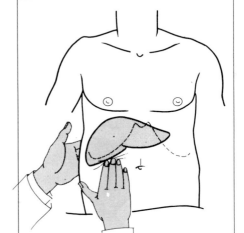

2

9 Try to determine the consistency of the liver tissue: is it soft or solid? Is the edge smooth or irregular? Do you feel any nodules?

10 Determine whether the edge of the liver is sharp (normal) or blunt.

B The gall bladder

The gall bladder is palpated in the same way as the liver.
●The gall bladder is often observed as an indentation in the liver at the level of the midclavicular line.

8.6 Palpation of the spleen

Purpose
To obtain an impression of the size and consistency of the spleen by palpation.

Procedure
1 Place your left hand on the left side of the patient's back on the lowermost rib. Press upward lightly with this hand.

2 Lay your right hand on the left side of the abdomen (Figures 1 and 2).

3 Ask the patient to exhale deeply.
 •When the spleen is enlarged you can feel its edge sliding under your fingers.

4 It is wise to repeat this palpation several times in succession, altering the position of your right hand each time.
 •This palpation is often facilitated by having the patient lie on the right side.

5 Attempt to estimate the size of the spleen.

6 Attempt to obtain an impression of the consistency of the spleen.

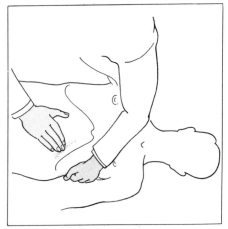

1

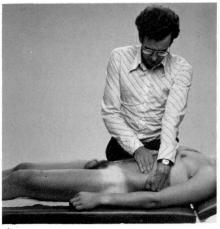

2

D 8.7 Palpation of other intra-abdominal organs and structures

Purpose

To obtain an impression of various abdominal organs and structures (size, shape, consistency, etc.) by palpation.

Procedure

A The kidneys

- Normally, the kidneys are not palpable.

1 Palpate the right kidney first: the procedure is the same as for the liver except that the right hand must be used a little more firmly and go deeper (Figures 1–3).

2 For kidney palpation, the right hand will have to make an upward movement.

3 Next, palpate the left kidney. The position of the left hand is lower in the lumbar region than for the spleen's palpation, and the right hand will be placed more medially and palpate upwards and deeply.

4 Lastly, perform a ballottement test:
   - place your hands in the palpation position on the right or left side,
   - with the fingers on the patient's back, make successive but firm flicking movements upward,
   - if the hand on the abdomen feels the flicking movement, renal ballottement is present.

B The bladder

1 Palpate from below the umbilicus, down towards the pubic symphysis.

2 Attempt to estimate the dimension and extension of the bladder (the circumference is convex).

3 Do not confuse with ascites, or a pregnant uterus.

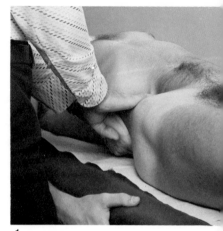

1

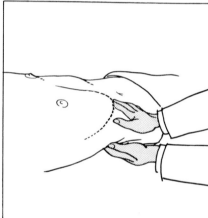

2

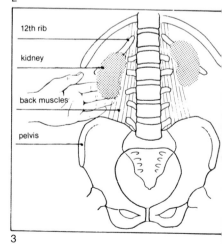

12th rib

kidney

back muscles

pelvis

3

C The aorta and other arteries

1 Palpate deeply, above the umbilicus and a little to the left of the midline.

2 You will then feel the pulsations of the aorta.

3 Both common iliac arteries can be palpated distal to this site.

D Other areas

1 Start in the epigastric region.

2 Palpate the abdomen systematically, with special attention to the course of the colon.

3 Palpate the region between the umbilicus and symphysis pubis carefully.

4 Do not be misled by a full bladder or a pregnant uterus.
   • Combine palpation findings with those obtained by inspection, auscultation, and percussion as you proceed.

D 8.8 Palpation of the groin

Purpose
To detect any abnormalities in the groin and inguinal area.

Procedure
1 Have the region completely exposed.

2 Make certain that your hands are warm.

3 Start by palpating the region with the tips of your fingers (Figure 1).

4 Look for swellings, signs of inflammation and any abnormalities in shape.

5 If you find a swelling, attempt to determine whether it is restricted to the scrotum, the neck of the scrotum, or the groin.
   ●Swelling of the lymph glands is usually multiple.

6 Attempt to determine the nature of any swelling.

7 Differentiate between a direct and an indirect inguinal hernia:
   - palpate the external inguinal ring by pressing diagonally upward in the scrotum with your little finger (Figure 2),
   - assess the size and consistency of the ring,
   - close the ring off with the little finger (or index finger),
   - ask the patient to press downwards or cough.
   ●A direct hernia can protrude (from posterior to anterior) between the deep epigastric artery and the edge of rectus muscle, an indirect inguinal hernia through the internal ring, obliquely through the inguinal canal.
   ●When the palpating finger is removed, the hernia may extrude (following the inguinal canal obliquely downwards).

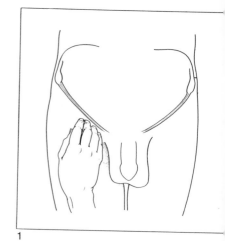

1

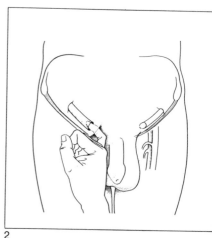

2

8 Distinguish between a retractile testis, an undescended testis, and testicular atrophy.

Purpose

To obtain an impression of the shape
and function of the anus and the rectum
as well as the nearby organs by means
of inspection and palpation.

Procedure

A Preparation

1 Tell the patient what you are about to do
and explain the purpose of the
examination.

2 Ask the patient to assume one of the
following positions:
- *knee−elbow position*
●advantage: favorable for inspection,
disadvantage: this position is
uncomfortable for a sick
patient; the high-lying
organs in the pelvic cavity
move away;
- *lateral recumbent position* (Figures 1
and 2)
●advantage: a comfortable position,
disadvantage: the anterior structures are
difficult to reach;
- *supine position* (Figure 3), a variation
of lithotomy position
●advantage: comfortable for the
patient; anterior structures
easily reached,
disadvantage: you will be impeded by
the buttocks, which will
prevent your finger from
reaching very high;

- *squatting position*
●advantage: the pelvic organs shift
slightly forward in the
abdomen,
disadvantage: the patient will probably
not be able to remain in
this position very long.

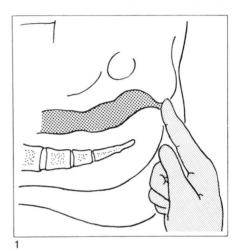

1

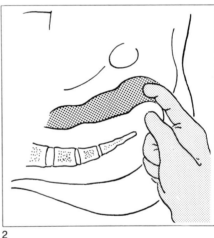

2

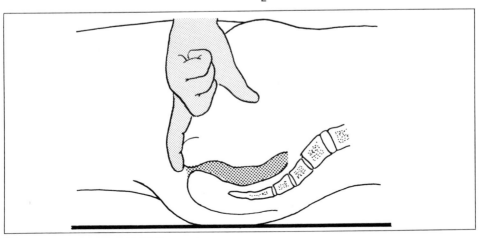

3

3 Make certain by percussion that the bladder is empty.

4 The distal part of the rectum must also be empty.

5 With a female patient, ask whether she has a contraceptive diaphragm, IUD or tampon in place.
  • Vaginal examination is performed before a rectal examination.

B Method

1 Inspect:
  - the perianal region: look for skin disorders, evidence of any fistula openings, swellings and ulcers;
  - the anus itself: spread the skin slightly and ask the patient to press gently and cautiously; look for internal and external hemorrhoids, fissures, fistula openings, mucous membrane prolapse, rectal prolapse or any secretions.

2 Reassure the patient by explaining what you are about to do and assuring that you will exercise great care.

3 The patient must breathe in and out comfortably.

4 Lubricate not only the gloved finger (not just the tip) but also the anus and its vicinity, especially the perianal hairs.

5 Lay the extended finger against the perineum with the tip at the entrance of the anus (Figure 1).

6 Press firmly with the extended finger and the sphincter muscle will relax to admit it.

7 Bend the finger inward over the anterior edge of the anus (Figure 2).

8 Pause a moment and tell the patient that the worst is over and that the anus should not be contracted.

9 The anus will then relax again and the finger will slide inward effortlessly.

10 Evaluate the tone of the sphincter muscle.

11 Let your finger slide further in and evaluate the condition of the surrounding rectal mucous membranes (hemorrhoids).

12 Palpate the prostate.

13 Palpate for the seminal vesicles above the prostate. In health, these are not palpable.

14 Palpate the area of the uterine cervix, the body of the uterus, and the adjacent tissues.

15 Ask the patient to press downwards: this lowers the contents of the abdominal and pelvic cavities and makes it easier to reach them.

16 Palpate the recto-uterine pouch or the rectovesical pouch (just reachable with the tip of the finger).

17 Palpate the bony structures of the pelvic region (promontory, lateral walls and sacrum).

18 Withdraw the finger gradually to permit repalpation of certain structures.

19 Check the glove for blood, mucus or pus.

9 Examination of the internal and external genitalia

Purpose
To obtain an impression of the male or female genitals by inspection and palpation.

Procedure

1 The patient is undressed below the waist.

2 The room and the examining hands should be warm.
 • Remember that many people find it very disagreeable to be naked.

3 Wear gloves.

4 By preference, the rectum and bladder should be empty.

5 Do not have the patient undressed longer than necessary.

6 Explain in detail what you are about to do.
 • In children and young girls, a full vaginal examination may only be possible under anesthesia.

7 Start with a full inspection of the secondary sexual characteristics and hair growth.

8 Continue with a detailed inspection of:
 - in a woman (Figure 1): the labia, vulva, vagina and cervix (a speculum will be required),
 - in a man (Figure 2): the penis and the scrotum.

9 Complete the examination with palpation of:
 in a woman: the labia majora and the internal genitals (vaginal examination),
 in a man: the testis, edipidymis, penis and prostate (rectal examination).

10 In a woman with gynecological complaints, rectal examination should be performed as well (D 8.9).

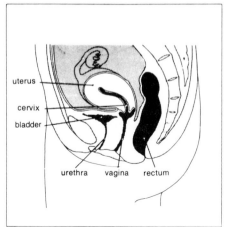

1

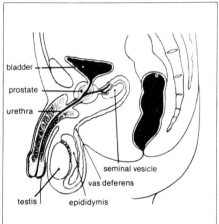

2

D 9.1　Secondary sexual characteristics

Purpose

To assess the degree of development of the secondary sexual characteristics as an evaluation of the advancement of puberty.

Procedure

1 The patient has undressed completely.

2 Determine the height and weight.

A　For young males

3 Determine the size of the testes.

4 Determine the size of the scrotum and penis.

5 Determine the stage of development of the pubic hair.
  ●There are five stages:
  - no pubic hair,
  - sparse growth of long, fine, non-curling hair, mainly at the base of the penis,
  - darker, coarser, loosely curling hair, over more of the pubic region,
  - hair resembling that of an adult but not yet fully distributed,
  - almost adult pattern: the upper margin is horizontal,
  Stage 6 is adult, showing extension along the linea alba and the abdominal skin.

6 Evaluate secondary hair growth elsewhere (armpits, upper lip, chin).

7 Note whether the voice has 'broken'.

8 Note the degree of breast development (the diameter of the nipple area; the areola becomes larger and the pigmentation deeper with maturity).

9 With these parameters, attempt to form an impression of the developmental stage.

B For young females

1 Evaluate the distribution of prepubertal
   fat.

2 Determine the stage of development of
   the breasts.
   ●There are five stages (see Figure):
   - the nipple is prominent,
   - prominence of the nipple, areola, and
     the breast itself,
   - increase of stage 2 but without
     distinct definition of shape,
   - the size of the breast increases,
     giving rise to a dome shape,
   - the secretory tissue and subcutaneous
     fat give an adult shape to the breast.

3 Determine the developmental stage of
   the pubic hair.
   ●There are five stages:
   - no pubic hair,
   - sparse growth of long, fine, non-curling
     hair, mainly along the labia majora.
   - darker, coarser, and loosely curled hair,
     over more of the pubic region,
   - hair resembling that of an adult but
     not yet fully distributed,
   - almost adult pattern: the upper margin
     is horizontal.

4 Note the size of the labia majora.

5 Note the size of the labia minora.

6 Ask when the menarche started.

7 With these parameters, attempt to form
   an impression of the developmental
   stage.

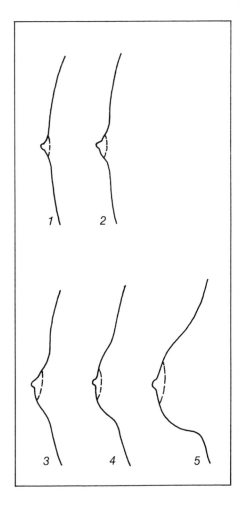

D 9.2 Inspection of the pubic hair

Purpose
To obtain an impression of the pattern of hair growth in the man/woman.

Procedure
1 The patient should undress completely.

2 Inspect systematically.

3 Start with the face.

4 Note hair distribution on chin and/or upper lip.

5 Then inspect the front and back of the thorax.

6 Ask the patient to raise the arms so you can see the hair in the armpits.

7 Inspect the hair on the abdomen.

8 Inspect the hair in the pubic region.
  •The pattern is not the same in men and women.

9 Inspect the peri-anal hair.

10 Inspect the hair in the groins, and on the upper legs and lower legs.

11 Note the density of the hair and the area covered.

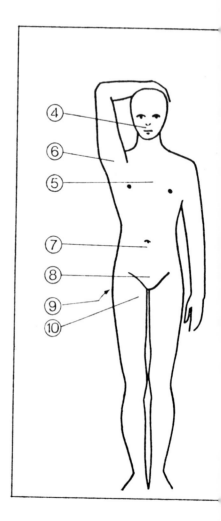

9.3 Inspection of the female external genitalia

Purpose
To obtain an impression of the development and condition of the female external genitals.

Procedure
1 The patient should undress to below the waist and lie on the examining table with her legs apart or in supports.

2 Inspection of the external genitals includes the hair, an assessment of the developmental stage and the condition of the skin.

3 Note the shape, size and condition of the labia majora on both sides.

4 Inspect the paraurethral ducts.

5 Inspect the orifice of the urethra.

6 Note the shape, size and condition of the clitoris.

7 Inspect the introitus, with special attention to the hymen or remnants of the hymen.

8 Next, inspect the labia minora (shape, size, color and condition).

9 Evaluate the perineum (inflammation, fistulas or swellings).

10 Ask the woman to press down so you can see whether, and if so how far, the vaginal walls and/or the cervix of the uterus descend.

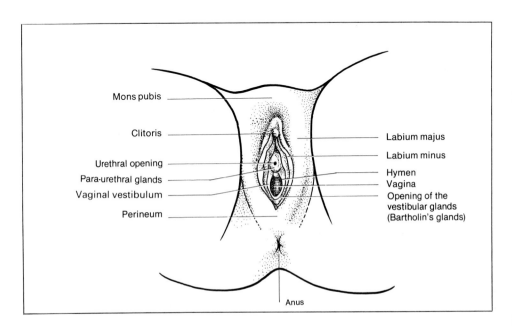

Mons pubis

Clitoris

Urethral opening

Para-urethral glands

Vaginal vestibulum

Perineum

Labium majus

Labium minus

Hymen

Vagina

Opening of the vestibular glands (Bartholin's glands)

Anus

D 9.4 Palpation of the labia majora

Purpose
To obtain an impression of the size, shape, and any abnormalities of the labia majora by palpation.

Procedure
1 Place the patient in the lithotomy position.

2 Put on a glove.

3 Take first the right and then the left labium majus between the thumb and the index and middle fingers (see Figure).

4 Palpate from top to bottom.

5 Watch for pressure pain and tumors or swellings.

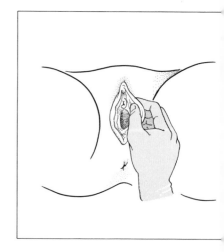

Purpose
Inspection of walls of the vagina and the cervix, if necessary with the establishment of patency of the vagina for diagnostic or therapeutic procedures (e.g. collection of material for smears, curettage, diathermy).

Procedure
1 The patient's body is exposed from the waist down and her knees are drawn up or her legs placed in supports.

2 Start by inspecting the external genitalia.

3 Spread the labia majora with the index finger and thumb of the gloved hand such that the labia minora separate.

4 With the right hand, introduce the closed speculum at a 45° angle into the opening of the vagina (Figure 1), exerting a small amount of pressure on the posterior wall (to spare the more sensitive and vulnerable anterior wall and particularly the urethra).

5 Advance the still-closed speculum into the vagina while rotating it 45° so that it lies transversely in the vagina.

6 Advance the closed speculum as far as possible, i.e. until it reaches the posterior fornix (Figure 2).

7 Open the speculum.

8 Manipulate the speculum until the cervix is visible (Figure 3).

9 Fix the open speculum in this position.

10 Continue the inspection of the contents of the vagina and the fornices, and note the colour, amount, consistency and odour of the secretions.

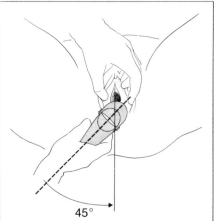

1

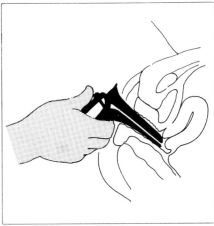

2

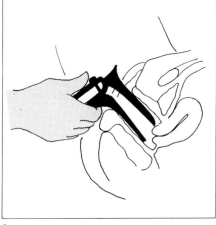

3

11 Then inspect the vaginal walls, their colour and condition, the lower parts, the surroundings and shape of the vaginal vault, and the shape, size and condition of the membranes surrounding the cervix.

12 Close the speculum, withdraw it slowly and carefully, and lay it aside.

13 While withdrawing it, look for any further abnormalities of the vagina.
   - The results of a gynaecological examination must always be interpreted in terms of the day of the cycle (e.g. clear cervical mucus on the 25th day is abnormal).

Purpose
To collect epithelial cells from the cervix.

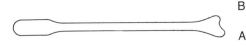

Procedure
- The preparation of a cervical smear is part of the gynaecological examination, and is done prior to a vaginal examination.

1 Adjust and insert the speculum; toilet of the vaginal opening is not performed.

2 Make certain you have good illumination.

3 Take a cervical spatula (Figure 1).

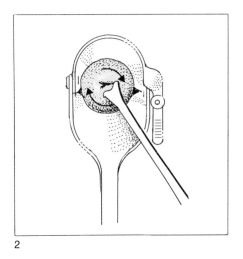

4 Place the leading tip (A) of the spatula in the vaginal orifice and up through the opened blades of the speculum.

5 Turn the spatula circularly (360°), so that tip B will scrape the cervix (Figure 2).

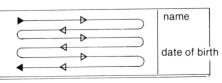

6 Spread the collected material in a thin, even layer on a glass slide (Figure 3).

7 Fix the material immediately with a fixative spray, or solution, and label the slide.

8 Make a cervical canal smear as well.

9 Use an applicator tipped with cotton wool moistened with saline.

10 Place the applicator in the cervical canal and rotate it against the wall without twisting it. (The applicator must not turn on its own axis).

11 Spread the material on a glass slide, fix it immediately, and label the slide.

12 Continue the gynaecological examination.

13 Send the smears to a cytology laboratory for evaluation.

D 9.7   Vaginal examination

Purpose

To evaluate the condition of the female internal genitals by a bimanual examination.

Procedure

- Vaginal examination is always performed after the speculum examination.
- The bladder must be empty.

1 The patient, who is undressed from the waist down, lies with her legs spread apart or in the leg supports.

2 Put on gloves.

3 Apply a lubricant to the second and third fingers of your right hand.

4 With the thumb and finger of the gloved left hand, spread the labia majora.
   - When the hymen is intact, an attempt should be made to introduce the index finger (for children, the little finger) into the vagina.

5 Bring the second and third fingers of the right hand together and in parallel with the opening of the vagina (antero-posteriorly) (Figure 1).

6 Apply light pressure upwards and towards the patient's back.

7 Advance the fingers as far as possible in the vagina.

8 Ask the patient to press down, so that you can check for any degree of prolapse of the uterus.

9 Palpate the fornices; determine the shape and depth.

10 Palpate the cervix.

11 Move the cervix back and forth gently (note the degree of mobility and whether any discomfort or pain is felt).

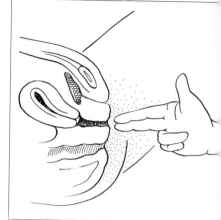

1

12 Place the flat left hand on the lower part of the abdominal wall and press inward gently above the symphysis.

13 Palpate the uterus between your hands (Figure 2).

14 Attempt to form an impression of the shape, size and mobility of the uterus and whether there is any pain on pressure.

15 Locate the right and left ovaries and the adjoining tissues to the uterus, bimanually.

16 Determine the size and shape and any tenderness or pain in these tissues.
• A normal ovary is often not palpable.

17 Next, evaluate the posterior fornix. Note fluid accumulation, resistance and tenderness.

18 Examine the deep pelvic tissues by pressing with the fingers at either side of the cervix.
• The tissues may show thickening or feel hard and tender.

19 Lastly, palpate the coccyx by moving the fingers backwards and downwards.

20 Withdraw the fingers carefully from the vagina.

21 Take off the gloves.

22 Vaginal and rectal examination can be combined to obtain a more precise examination of the perineum, and the rectovaginal areas. The index finger can be introduced rectally, and the thumb vaginally.

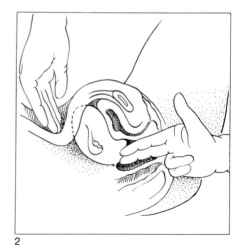
2

Purpose
To obtain, by inspection, an impression of the anatomy and any abnormalities of the male external genitalia.

Procedure
1 Make sure you have good illumination.

2 Inspect the patient both standing and lying down.

3 Inspect systematically.

4 Start with the pubic region.

5 Note the color and distribution of the hair.

6 Look for swellings in the inguinal area.

7 Note any skin lesions, swellings or parasites in the pubic region.

8 Then inspect the penis.

9 Inspect the skin of the penis.

10 Inspect the foreskin. Ask the patient to retract it over the glans. Note whether it can be retracted and whether there are ulcerations, smegma, or signs of inflammation (Figure 1).

11 Inspect the glans, with special attention to the corona.

12 Next, inspect the urethral opening.

13 Note the shape, size, and location.

14 Then inspect the scrotum.

15 Inspect the skin of the scrotum (for any swollen sebaceous glands, other swellings, inflammation or parasites).

16 Inspect the back of the scrotum by lifting it up (Figure 2).

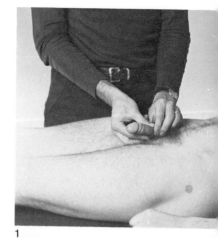

1

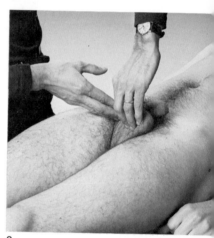

2

17 In addition, attempt to obtain an impression of the contents of the scrotum by inspection.
 • Normally, the left testis hangs lower than the right.

Palpation of the penis

Purpose
To obtain an impression of the shape
and any abnormalities of the penis by
palpation.

Procedure
1 The patient may be seated or lying
   down.

2 Palpate the penis from the pelvic end
   outwards.

3 The shaft can be evaluated best by
   taking it between your thumb and your
   index and middle fingers (see Figure).

4 Note any pain brought about by
   pressure, or tenderness, indurations and
   the shape and size.

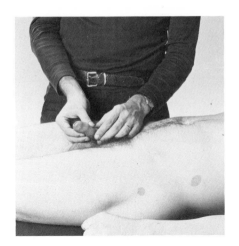

D 9.10 Palpation of the scrotum

Purpose

To obtain an impression of the organs in the scrotum by palpation.

Procedure

1 Palpate the skin of the scrotum first.

2 For this purpose, take hold of a fold of the skin between your thumb and your index and middle fingers (Figure 1).

3 Look in particular for any swellings.

4 Take hold of the testicle in the same way.

5 Palpate the testicles systematically from the upper pole to the lower.

6 Note the size, shape and consistency and sensitivity to gentle pressure.

7 Identify the spermatic cord and palpate it from the epididymis to the inguinal ring.

8 Look for any swellings.

9 Palpate the epididymis.
 ●Any swelling found in the scrotum must be investigated further by transillumination.

10 For this purpose, darken the room.

11 Use a small torch and direct the light beam through the swelling from behind (Figure 2).

12 Note whether the light shines through.
 ●Light can pass through serous fluid but not through blood or solid tissue.

13 Lastly, palpate the inguinal canal with your little finger (D 8.8).

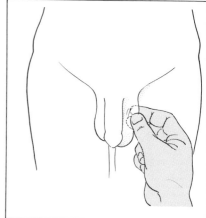

1

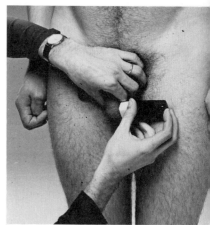

2

0 Examination of a pregnant woman

Purpose
To estimate the progress of a
pregnancy.

Procedure

A General conditions

1 Tell the patient what you are about to do
and why.

2 Ask her to lie down, by preference on a
firm surface.

3 The lower part of the body should be
exposed.

4 She should lie with her legs flat or with
the knees raised such that the legs stay
in position without her having to use
(abdominal) muscles to keep them in
place (see Figure).

5 The patient's bladder should be empty.

6 Provide adequate warmth (warm hands,
warm examination couch and warm
stethoscope).

B The examination

7 Weigh the patient.

8 Measure the blood pressure with the
patient sitting or lying.

9 Test the urine for protein and glucose.

10 Start the inspection with the abdomen
and the external genitals.

11 Estimate the level of the fundus by
means of inspection, percussion, and
palpation.

12 Attempt to determine the position of the
fetus.

13 Listen to the fetal heart sounds.

14 Check for edema

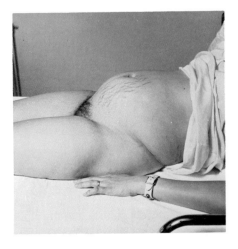

15 At the first examination during the
pregnancy, assess the internal pelvic
organs and cavity (D 9.7 and D 10.2).

16 Ask the patient to dress.

17 Record your findings.

D 10.1 Inspection of the vulva and vagina

Purpose
To evaluate the changes in the vulva and vagina associated with pregnancy.

Procedure
• This examination is part of the gynecological examination.

1 Spread the labia minora with the thumb and index finger.

2 Inspect the mucous membranes of the vulva and vagina (see Figure).
• In a pregnant woman the tissues are slightly edematous and the mucous membrane colour is bluish−red.

3 Look for any abnormal changes (e.g. varicosities).

4 Then insert the speculum.

5 Note the color of the vaginal walls while doing so.

6 Note the shape of the cervical opening.
• In nullipara the shape is round, in multipara it is split shaped.

7 Remove the speculum and continue with the vaginal examination (D 9.7).

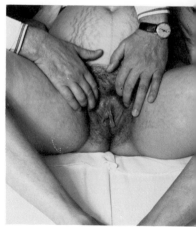

1

.2 Palpation of the pelvic cavity

Purpose
To obtain an impression of the lower part of the pelvic cavity by internal examination.

Procedure
1 The patient is undressed from the waist down and lies on her back with the legs apart or supported.

2 Perform the vaginal examination (D 9.7).

3 Attempt to reach the promontory to determine whether the pelvis is narrow.
  ● When the pelvis is normal the promontory is usually impossible to reach.

4 If you can reach the promontory, measure the distance from it to the lower edge of the symphysis (normally about 12.5 cm; Figure 1).

5 A rough estimate of the width of the inlet to the pelvis can be obtained by palpating to either side, to reach the innominate arch.
  ● If this edge cannot be followed in the posterior third, the inlet is sufficiently wide (Figure 2).

6 Palpate the inner side of the base of the pelvis on the right and left to find out whether the ischial tuberosities project, and also the sacrospinal ligament for mid-pelvic contraction (Figure 3).

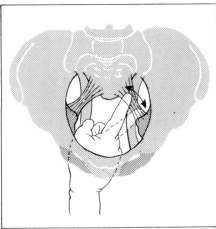

1

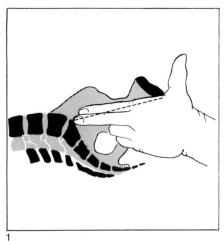

2

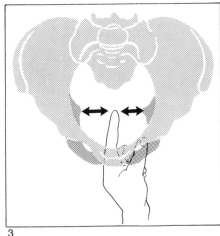

3

7 Feel whether the arch is sufficiently wide (more than 90°) or too narrow (less than 90°): (i.e. pelvic outlet contraction), by placing the knuckles of your hand between the ischial tuberosities (Figure 4).
●Normally, four knuckles will fit.

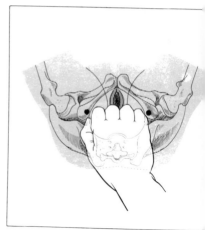

4

0.3 Determination of the position of the uterine fundus

Purpose
To obtain an impression of the shape and size of the uterus by inspection, percussion, and palpation.

Procedure
● This examination is part of the gynecological examination.

1. Attempt to obtain an impression of the shape of the uterus by inspection.

2. Attempt to obtain an impression of the position of the uterus (Figure 1).

3. Note any evidence of fetal movements.
   ● Gentle percussion is particularly helpful from the fourth month of pregnancy.

4. Percuss the abdomen.

5. Determine, by percussion, the boundaries of the uterus (Figure 2).

6. Palpate with the hand flat; in particular, avoid pressing on the abdomen with your fingers (this is very unpleasant for the woman, and therefore, her abdominal muscles will contract).

7. Palpate with a flat hand to determine the shape of the uterus.

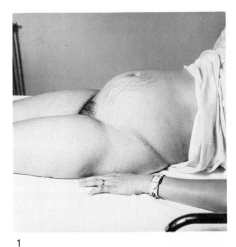

1

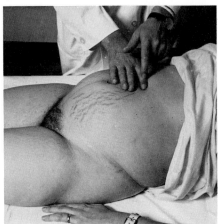

2

8 For this purpose, lay your hands to the left and right of the fundus (Figure 3).

9 If necessary, gently bring the uterus into the midline.

10 Now determine the height of the uterus relative to the symphysis pubis and umbilicus, or to the umbilicus and xiphoid process, at the lower end of the sternum.

11 Record the height of the fundus in relation to these points.

12 Correlate the height of the uterus with the duration of the pregnancy.

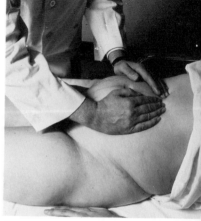

3

13 You can also use a tapemeasure to measure the distance between the upper edge of the symphysis and the upper edge of the fundus (over the umbilicus).
●The period of amenorrhea should be equal to the number of centimetres plus 4.

14 Record your findings.

Purpose
To determine the position of the fetus in the uterus.

Procedure
● This determination is part of the obstetric examination in any pregnancy of a duration of 24 weeks or more.

1 Stand to the right of the patient facing her.

2 Palpate with both hands flat. Avoid pressing your fingers into her abdomen (because this is unpleasant and the abdominal muscles will contract).

3 With both hands, palpate to determine the shape of the uterus.

4 Start close to the lowest rib.

5 By the application of light pressure you will feel the fetus (Figure 1).

6 Attempt to determine which part of the fetus is in the fundus (i.e. uppermost).
● An irregular shape is another part of the fetus, e.g. breech; a round shape is the head.
● The breech is not susceptible to ballottement but the head is.

7 Next, slide your hands along the sides of the uterus in the direction of the symphysis.

8 On one side you will feel a firm consistent resistance, which is the back; on the other side you will feel irregular small lumps, which are the arms and legs (Figure 2).

9 Place your right hand above the symphysis with the thumb on one side of the projection and the four fingers on the other side (Figures 3 and 4).

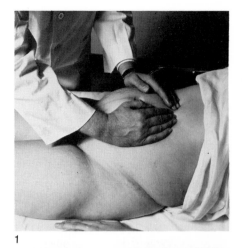

1

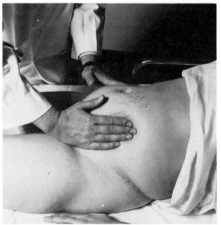

2

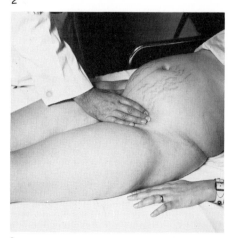

3

10 Make gentle movements from side to
    side.
    ● If the projecting part is an undescended
      vertex, you will feel it moving back and
      forth like a hard round ball: i.e.
      ballottement.

11 Now turn towards the patient's feet.

12 Place your hands on each side of the
    lowest part of the uterus (Figure 5).

13 The patient should draw up her knees
    so that her abdominal muscles are
    completely relaxed.

14 Attempt to determine which part of the
    fetus is in this area by palpating the
    projecting part during exhalation,
    pressing lightly on the uterus. Note
    ballottement here too.

15 Determine by palpation which part of
    the vertex still lies above the pelvic inlet.

16 Record the position of the fetus.

17 Continue the examination with
    auscultation of the fetal heart sounds.

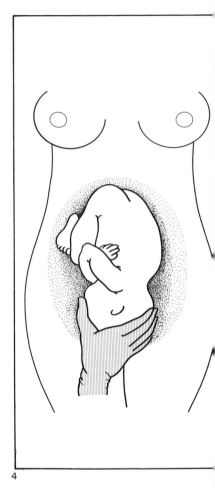

4

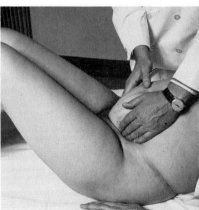

5

10.5 Auscultation of the fetal heart sounds

Purpose
To obtain an impression of the heart action of the fetus and location of the point of maximum intensity of the sounds, as a parameter for the determination of the position of the fetus.

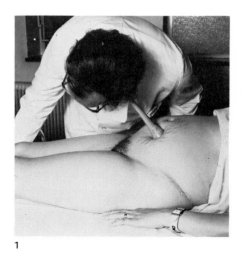

Procedure
● Fetal heart sounds cannot be heard before the 18th week.

1 For this examination make use of a fetal stethoscope.

2 Place the stethoscope on the patient's abdomen.

1

3 Lay your ear on the other end of the stethoscope (Figure 1).

4 Apply a small amount of pressure to the abdomen.

5 Listen to the fetal heart action.
 ● This action is rapid (120−160 beats per minute).

6 Make certain that you do not confuse the maternal aorta sounds with the fetal heart sounds (by simultaneously checking the pulse at the patient's wrist).

7 You will often have to search for the place where the fetal heart sounds are the most distinct.
 ● This is usually the place where the anterior shoulder is situated.

8 Record the frequency in number of beats per minute.

D 11   Examination of the trunk

Purpose
To obtain an impression of the shape
and functioning of the vertebral column.

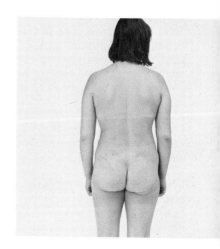

Procedure
• Examination of the back is often part of
the assessment of muscular function.

1 The patient should be naked.

2 The examination is performed with the
patient at rest, in motion, and in the
standing, sitting and supine positions.

3 Compare the right and left sides
throughout.

4 Remember that the back also casts its
"shadow" on the front of the patient's
body.

5 Start with inspection of the trunk while
the patient stands at ease.

6 Ask the patient to perform a number of
movements.

7 Note to what extent this can be done
and how it is done.

8 Next, palpate the back while the patient
stands erect.

9 Then palpate while the patient performs
a number of movements.

10 Evaluate the effective functioning of the
back.

11 In your evaluations, take into
consideration the findings concerning
the pelvis, knees and feet.

12 Lastly, perform a neurological
examination of the trunk.

Purpose
To obtain an impression of the shape of
the back and the position and posture in
which the thorax and pelvis are held.

Procedure
1 The patient stands with the feet a little
apart, at ease and relaxed (Figure 1).

2 Start by forming a general impression of
the patient and posture.

3 Attempt to form an impression of the
patient's nutritional status and general
health (obesity, development of the
musculature, extent of skin folds,
protrusion of the ribs).

4 Next, inspect the back.

5 Inspect the skin (discoloration,
inflammation, pathological hair growth,
scars and any difference in skin folds
between right and left sides).

6 Look for any swellings.

7 Inspect the musculature (increase or
decrease of circumference).

8 Evaluate the natural curvatures of the
spine (Figure 2):
- cervical lordosis,
- thoracic kyphosis,
- lumbar lordosis.
Inspect the patient from the front and
from both sides.

9 Then look for scoliosis (convex toward
the right or left).

10 Note whether the scoliosis has been
compensated for. For this purpose, see
whether a straight line from the foramen
magnum passes between the buttocks
and ends exactly between the feet.

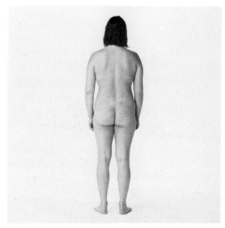

1

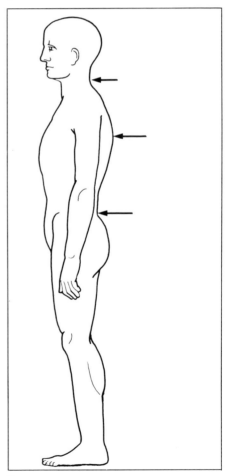

2

11 Note whether the spinous processes lie in a straight line (Figure 3).

12 Next, look for any torsion of the vertebral column (position of shoulders relative to hips).

13 Look for any kyphosis.

14 Note any postural anomalies.
- Postural anomalies can be distinguished from anatomical abnormalities on the basis of examination during movement. A compensatory scoliosis is a postural anomaly, a permanent kyphosis is an anatomical abnormality.
- Postural anomalies can be corrected.

15 Note deformities of the trunk.
- These can be a reflection of abnormalities of the vertebral column.

16 Therefore, note:
- the position of the shoulders, malformations of the thorax, the contours of the trunk (Figure 3),
- any differences in the spaces between the resting arms at the side and the trunk and the armpit contact.

17 In the lumbar region, pay special attention to the paralumbar musculature and indications of spina bifida (a pit in the skin or tuft of hair above the natal cleft or between the buttocks).

18 Continue the examination with inspection of the thorax.

19 Here, pay special attention to (Figure 4):
- any asymmetry of the thorax, or
- asymmetric respiratory excursions,
- the development of the thorax,
- congenital and acquired malformations,
- anomalies in the shape of the sternum.

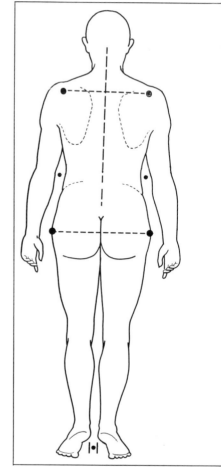

3

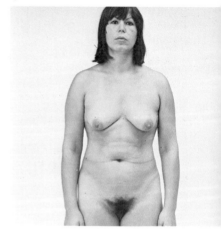

4

20 End the examination with an examination of the abdomen and pelvis.

21 Note (Figure 5):
- the shape of the abdomen,
- the symmetry of the abdomen,
- the position of the hips,
- hernias (epigastric, umbilical, inguinal, femoral or in scar tissue).

22 Pay special attention to the position the pelvis is held in, and any tilting.

23 For this, place your index fingers on the iliac crests and determine whether one is lower than the other (Figure 6).

24 Then determine whether this, or any scoliosis, can be corrected by the pressing up of one or other heel.

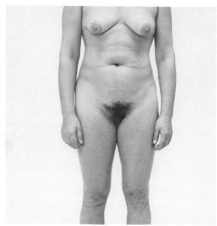

5

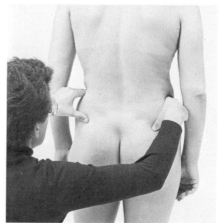

6

D 11.2 Palpation of the trunk

Purpose
To obtain information about the shape of the trunk and any anomalies in this region by palpation.

Procedure

1 Start by palpating with the patient standing.

2 Place your thumb and index finger to the right and left of the spinous process (Figure 1).

3 Now let your fingers slide down along the vertebral column while exerting an even pressure on the back.

4 Note any deviations of the vertebral column.

5 Look for prominence of one of the processes or the absence of a process.

6 Then detect any discomfort in the vertebral column by percussing the individual vertebrae (Figure 2).

7 Detect pressure pain between the vertebrae by:
  - asking the patient to stand on tiptoe and then let the heels "fall",
  - put your hands on the patient's head or shoulders and press downward forcefully, which increases the pressure on the vertebral column (Figure 3).

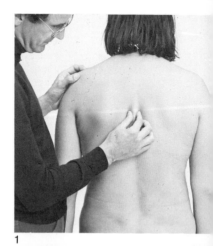

1

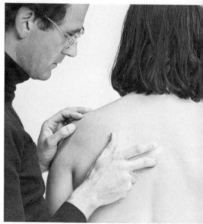

2

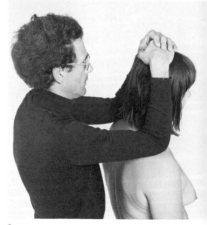

3

8   Then ask the patient to lie prone with the head turned sideways (by preference without a pillow) and the arms stretched beside the body on the examining table; the patient must be completely relaxed (Figure 4).

9   With the back of your hand, check the skin for differences in temperature (Figure 5).

10 Palpate the muscles of the back (atrophy, excessive tension, pressure pain or any swellings).

11 Then palpate the vertebral column:
    - the spinous processes,
    - the interspinal ligaments,
    - as well as the iliac spines.

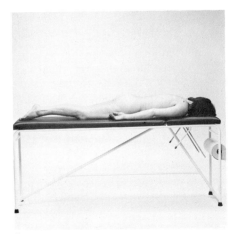

4

12 Palpate the sacro-iliac joint (swelling, elevated temperature, painfulness; Figure 6).

13 Palpate the gluteal musculature.

14 Ask the patient to lie on one side.

15 Palpate the skin and muscles of the thorax and abdomen (temperature differences, swellings, etc.).

16 Palpate the sternum and its joints.

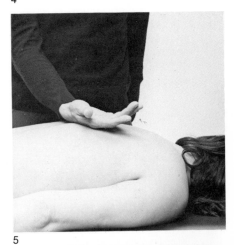

5

17 Press the palm of your hands against the sternum, thus compressing the thorax inwards (Figure 7); note whether this is painful.

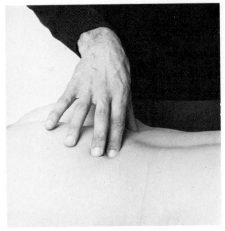

6

18 Next, palpate the ribs; check for defects, swellings and any pain.

19 Continue the examination with palpation of the abdominal wall, paying special attention to the musculature and the presence of any swellings or hernias.

20 Then palpate the bony part of the pelvis, with special attention to any pain at pressure on the symphysis (Figure 8).

21 Examine the sacro-iliac joints by lateral compression of the hips (Figure 9).

22 Lastly, palpate the coccyx (any excessive movements and pain).

23 If necessary, perform a rectal examination.

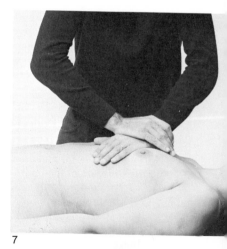
7

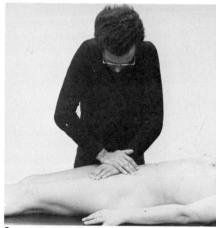
8

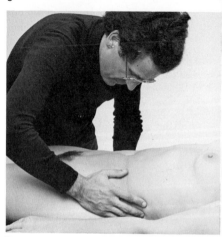
9

11.3 Inspection of the active movements of the trunk

Purpose
To obtain an impression of the capacity of the back for active movement.

Procedure

1 The patient should stand with the feet spread apart, at ease and relaxed.

2 Ask the patient to bend over (anteflexion) without bending the knees and see whether this movement is performed smoothly and sufficiently far without any rigidity (Figure 1).

3 Evaluate dorsiflexion as well (extension).

4 Evaluate lateral flexion (right and left; Figure 2).

5 Evaluate rotation after fixation of the hips by having the patient sit down (Figure 3).

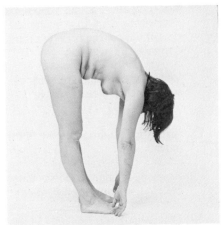

1

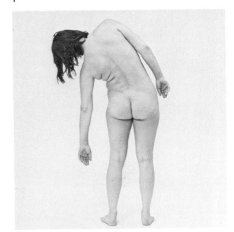

2

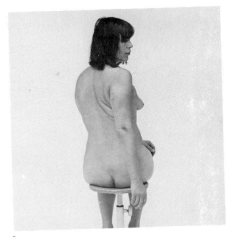

3

6 Ask the patient to raise the arms, and inspect the back to see whether any deformities of the back are thus corrected (Figure 4).

7 While the patient's arms are raised, see whether the scapulae move symmetrically.

8 Note any restrictions of all of these movements.

9 Note any changes in the position of the vertebral column.

10 Take note of any pain felt by the patient.

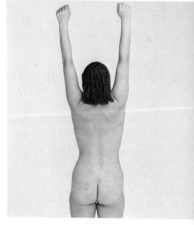

4

11 Important information can be obtained by watching the patient walk. Pay special attention to changes in the shape of the back and the movements of the hips.

12 Lastly, perform specific trunk function tests (D 11.6).

11.4 Palpation of the moving trunk

Purpose
To obtain an impression of the course
of the trunk movements.

Procedure
1 Palpate successively:
   - while standing, flexion and extension
     movements (Figure 1),
   - while sitting, rotational and lateral
     flexion movements (Figure 2),
   - while lying prone, extension
     movements.

2 Throughout, palpate the spinous
  processes of the vertebrae (to detect
  any pain, crepitation, or swellings).

3 Pay special attention to the musculature
  (note the tone, any pain or spasm and
  the degree of contraction).

4 Palpate the respiratory excursions (B 7).

5 Pay special attention to the sacro-iliac
  joints.

6 In this connection note any pain or
  swelling.

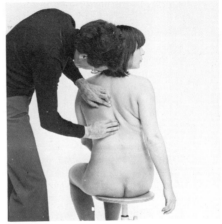

1

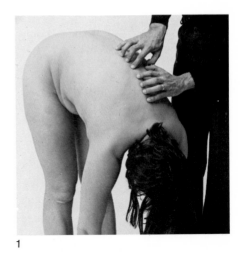

2

D 11.5 Passive movements of the trunk

Purpose
To obtain an impression of the passive movements of the trunk.

Procedure

1 Ask the patient to stand.

2 Flex the patient's back by pushing the head forward and downward with one hand and holding the hips back with the other hand (Figures 1 and 2).

3 Note whether, and if so to what extent, this is possible and how this movement occurs.

4 Pay special attention to any fixations or rigidity in the vertebral column.

5 Measure flexion extension by placing your thumb and index finger at the site of the lumbosacral joint and 10 cm above that point, respectively.
 ●The resulting distance between the two fingers should amount to about 15 cm.

6 Next, perform extension of the trunk.

7 With the patient seated, perform the rotational and lateral flexion movements (Figure 3).

8 Note whether deviations in the position of the vertebral column are corrected by specific movements.
 ●You can probably obtain more information when the patient is lying supine or prone; it is easier for the patient to relax in these positions.

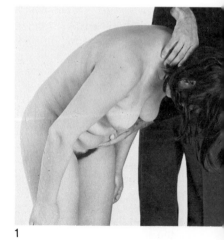

1

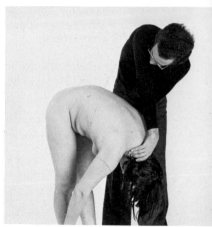

2

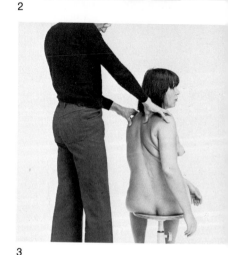

3

Purpose
To obtain information about the
functioning of the trunk by means of
specific tests.

Procedure

A

1 Stand behind the patient.

2 Ask the patient to bend one leg at the
hip and knee ('stork' position; see
Figure).

3 Note what the pelvis does.
  • If the pelvis slants toward the side of
  the raised leg there is weakness in the
  power of the gluteal muscles.

B

1 Ask the patient to stand straight with
the legs together.

2 Scoliosis of the spine due to a
difference in the length of the legs can be
corrected by eliminating this difference.

3 To eliminate the difference place blocks
differing in thickness under the short
leg.

4 Estimate how many centimetres the
heel must be raised to correct the
scoliosis.

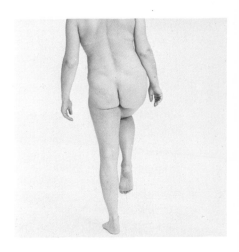

D 12 Examination of the arm

Purpose
To obtain an impression of the shape and functioning of the arm.

Procedure

1 Ask the patient to undress to the waist.

2 Start with inspection, and do this systematically.

3 Remember that four sides must receive attention.

4 Compare right and left at each step.

5 Start with inspection of the shoulder.

6 Inspect the shoulder while the arm rests relaxed at the patient's side,

7 and during movement of the shoulder.

8 Next, palpate the resting and moving shoulder.

9 Evaluate the functioning of the shoulder.

10 Continue the examination with inspection, palpation, and function−evaluation of the shoulder.

11 Examine the wrist and the hand in the same way.

12 If necessary, examine the peripheral circulation.

13 If necessary, measure the circumference of the arms.

14 Lastly, perform a neurological examination of the arm (C 4).

12.1 Examination of the peripheral circulation of the arm

Purpose

To obtain an impression of the quality of the peripheral vascular system, i.e. the peripheral circulation.

Procedure

1 The arms should be completely exposed.

2 Compare right and left at each step.

3 Record your findings systematically.

4 Start with an inspection of the skin. Pay attention to:
   - color changes at rest,
   - color changes on elevation of the limbs: with the arms raised above the head, feel whether the pulse in the wrist disappears, note color changes in this position, and note color changes after the patient has made a fist 20 times,
   - color changes when the hands become cool,
   - trophic disturbances accompanying skin changes (e.g. ulceration, infections),
   - visible arterial pulsations,
   - hyperhydrosis.

5 Continue the examination with palpation. Palpate:
   - the temperature of both arms to detect any differences,
   - the subclavian, brachial (Figure 1), radial (Figure 2), and ulnar arteries,
   - note the condition of the walls of these arteries (normally not palpable, the margins imprecise, the vessel easily compressed and elastic),
   - evaluate the pulse wave.

6 Next, perform auscultation and note:
   - the number of sounds per beat,
   - vascular murmurs,
   - the regularity of the rhythm,
   - equality of the pulsation.

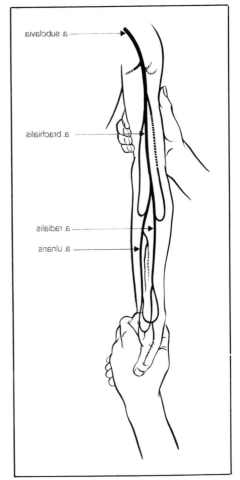

1

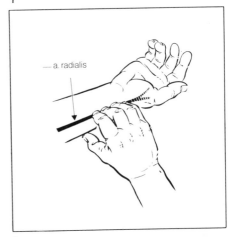

2

D 12.2 Measurement of the circumference of the arm

Purpose
To obtain an impression of any atrophy or hypertrophy by measurement of the circumference of the upper arm.

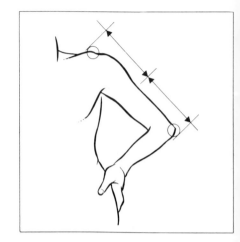

Procedure

1 The upper arm must be entirely exposed.

2 Ask the patient to put the hands on the hips.

3 Find the midpoint between the acromion and the olecranon (see Figure).

4 Mark this point.

5 With a tape measure passing over this point, measure the perpendicular to the longitudinal axis of the arm.

6 Measure the circumference to an accuracy of 0.1 cm.

7 Compare the right and left arm.

D 13 Examination of the shoulder girdle

Purpose
To obtain an impression of the shape
and functioning of the shoulders.

Procedure

1 Ask the patient to undress to the waist.

2 Perform your examination with the
patient sitting or standing.

3 Examine the front and back and do not
forget the sides.

4 Start with the inspection of the resting
shoulder.

5 Ask the patient to make a number of
movements.

6 Evaluate the degree to which, and how
these movements are performed.

7 Palpate the resting and moving shoulder.

8 Palpate the armpit as well.

9 Evaluate the mobility (and immobility) of
the shoulder.

10 Compare right and left.

11 Complete the examination with
measurements, and neurological and
vascular examinations.

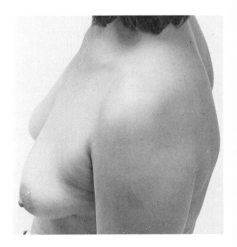

D 13.1 Inspection of the shoulders at rest

Purpose
To obtain an impression of the
shoulders by inspection.

Procedure

1 The patient should stand with arms
relaxed (Figure 1).

2 Inspect the shoulders from the front,
back and sides.

3 Inspect the skin over the joint
(discoloration, scars).

4 Note the contours of the shoulder
(flattening, sagging, swelling).

5 Note the position of the arm, especially
the contact between the arm and the
wall of the thorax at the armpit and the
outline of the space between the arm
and the body, on both sides (Figure 2).

6 Note the appearance of the arm
(increase or decrease of size); if
necessary, measure the circumference
of the upper arm (D 12.2).

7 Note the position of the scapula in
relation to the vertebral column
(Figure 3).

8 Inspect the surrounding areas of the
shoulder, including:
 - the clavicle,
 - the acromion,
 - the infra- and supraclavicular fossa,
 - the sternoclavicular joint,
 - the sternum,
 - the acromioclavicular joint.

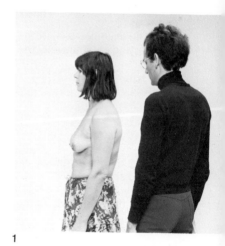

1

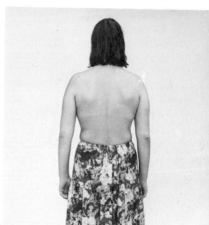

2

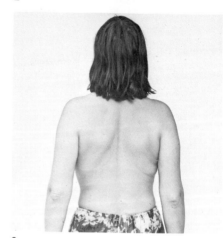

3

Purpose

To obtain an impression of the shape of
the shoulders by palpation.

Procedure

1 The patient is seated with relaxed arms
   resting by the side.

2 Palpate the skin over the joint
   (temperature, mobility and any swelling;
   Figure 1).

3 Palpate the muscles around the joint
   and their sites of attachment (tone, pain
   and resistance; Figure 2).

4 Palpate the joint capsule, starting at the
   front and proceeding along the edge of
   the deltoid muscle (to detect any
   swelling, pain or tenderness).

5 Palpate the articulation of the joints:
   - lay your flat hand deep in the armpit
     (Figure 3),
   - palpate the head of the humerus in the
     glenoid cavity,
   - rotate the humerus passively with the
     elbow flexed, and at the same time
     palpate the head of the humerus,
   - attempt to palpate the edge of the
     glenoid cavity.

6 Palpate the armpit (D 7.17).

7 Palpate the bony parts of the joint, e.g.
   the head of the humerus, the tubercle of
   the humerus, the acromion, the scapula,
   the coracoid process, and the clavicle
   (note pain, crepitation, dislocation and
   abnormal shape).

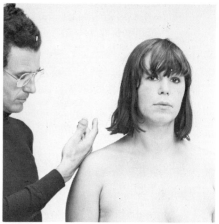

1

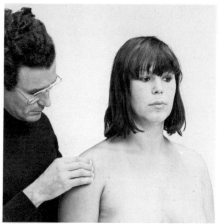

2

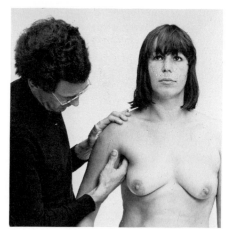

3

D 13.3 Inspection of the active movements of the shoulder

Purpose
To obtain an impression of the range of mobility of the shoulders by means of inspection.

Procedure

1 The patient is asked to stand with the arms stretched above the head.

2 Inspect successively the active movements:
 - anteflexion,
 - retroflexion,
 - abduction,
 - adduction,
 - inward and outward rotation (with bent elbows); Figures 1−6.

3 Evaluate the ease with which these movements are performed.

4 Note any restriction of these movements.

5 Note any positional changes relative to the vertebral column.

6 Note whether any pain is felt.

7 Lastly, evaluate the power of the movements by asking the patient to perform them while you attempt to apply restraint with your hands.

8 Do not forget to inspect the dorsal aspect. Pay particular attention to the movements of the scapulae.

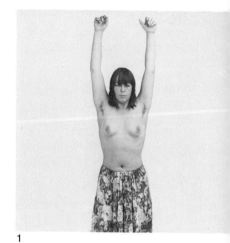

1

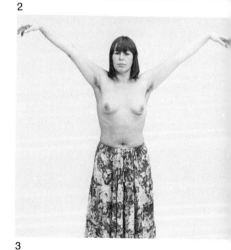

2

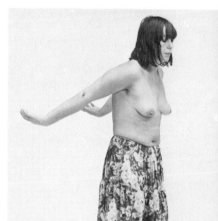

3

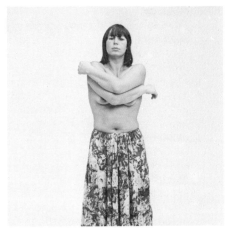

4

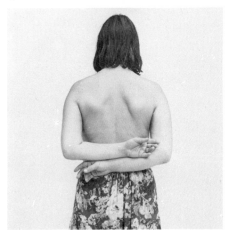

5

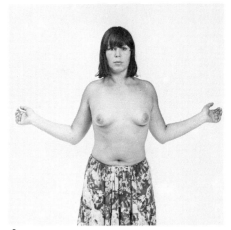

6

D 13.4 Palpation of the moving shoulder

Purpose
To obtain an impression of the shoulder movements.

Procedure

1 Ask the patient to perform the shoulder movements.

2 Place the palm of your hand on the patient's shoulder (Figure 1).

3 Note crepitations, resistance, and the degree of mobility (Figure 2).

4 With your finger tips, palpate the course of the various movements in the armpits.

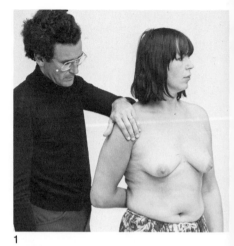

1

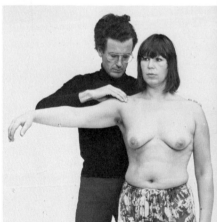

2

3.5 Passive movements of the shoulder

Purpose
To obtain an impression of the range of movement of the shoulders.

Procedure
1 Place one of your hands on the patient's shoulder.

2 With your other hand, grasp the upper arm at the level of the elbow.

3 Perform the following movements:
   - anteflexion,
   - retroflexion,
   - abduction (Figure 1),
   - adduction (Figure 2),
   - inward and outward rotation.

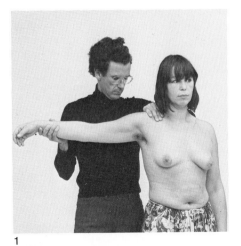

1

4 Evaluate whether, and if so to what extent, each of these movements can be performed.

5 Evaluate the course of each movement.

6 Pay special attention to:
   - exaggerated or limited mobility,
   - blocking,
   - cogwheel phenomenon,
   - resistance,
   - crepitation,
   - pain.

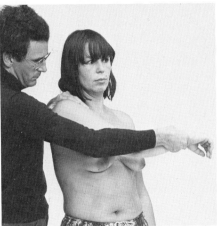

2

D 14   Examination of the elbow

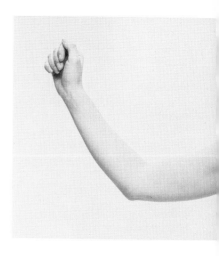

Purpose
To obtain an impression of the shape
and functioning of the elbow.

Procedure
1 Ask the patient to undress to the waist.

2 Have the patient stand while you
  perform the examination.

3 Examine all four sides throughout.

4 Start with inspection of the relaxed
  elbow.

5 Then ask the patient to perform
  movements with the elbow.

6 Judge whether, and if so to what extent,
  these movements are possible.

7 Then palpate the elbow at rest and in
  movement.

8 Evaluate the range of mobility of the
  elbow.

9 Compare left and right.

10 Lastly, perform a neurological
   examination and examine the peripheral
   circulation.

14.1 Inspection of the elbow at rest

Purpose
To obtain an impression of the shape of the elbow joint.

Procedure
1 The patient stands with the arms resting relaxed or with relaxed flexion (90°) of the elbow (Figures 1 and 2).

2 Inspect the elbow from the front, from the sides, and from the back in both the straight and flexed positions.

3 Inspect the skin over the joint (discoloration, scars).

4 Note the contours of the elbow (flattening or swelling).
 ●Take as reference points the line for the extended arm in relation to the trunk, and for the flexed arm.

5 Note the position of the arm, and in particular that of the lower arm relative to the upper arm.

6 Note the appearance of both the upper and the lower arm (increase or decrease in size) and if appropriate, measure the circumference.

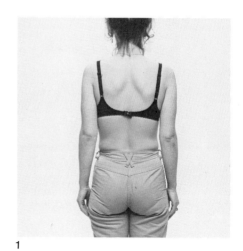

1

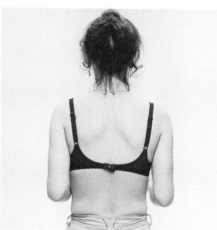

2

D 14.2 Palpation of the elbow at rest

Purpose
To obtain an impression of the shape of the elbow by palpation.

Procedure
1 The patient stands with relaxed arms resting at the side and then with the elbow flexed to 90°.

2 Palpate the skin over the joint (temperature, mobility, swellings).

3 Palpate the muscles around the elbow (tone, pain, any firm swellings).

4 Palpate the joint capsule of the elbow, using a dorsal approach (Figures 1 and 2).

5 Palpate the ligaments of the elbow joint (lateral ulnar and lateral radial ligaments).

6 Next, palpate the bony parts of the elbow.

7 Pay special attention to shape and circumference and also to any sensations of pain.

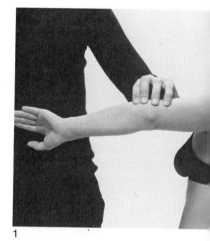

1

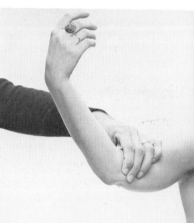

2

4.3 Inspection of the active movements of the elbow

Purpose
To obtain an impression of the functioning of the elbow by inspection.

Procedure
1 The patient stands with arms stretched or bent at the elbow.

2 Inspect successively the active movements:
   - flexion and extension (Figures 1 and 2),
   - pro- and supination (elbow flexed 90°) and upper arm pressed against the body (Figures 3 and 4).

3 Note whether these movements are performed smoothly.

4 Note any restrictions to these movements.

5 Note any pain.

6 Assess the strength of all movements by asking the patient to perform them while you apply restraint.

7 Perform the 'chair test'. Ask the patient to lift a chair by the back, first with pronated forearm (extensors) and then with supinated forearm (flexors).

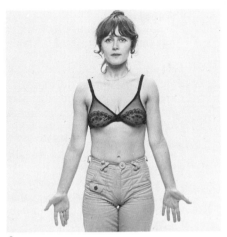

2

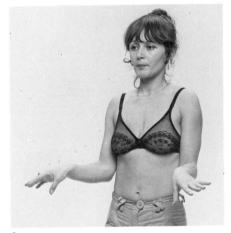

3

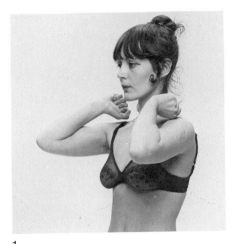

1

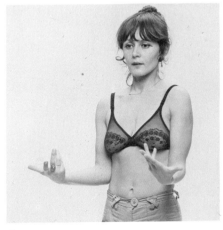

4

D 14.4 Palpation of the moving elbow

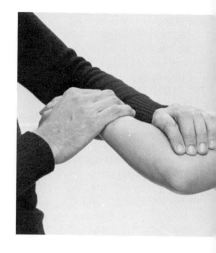

Purpose
To obtain an impression of the
functioning of the elbow by palpation.

Procedure
1 Palpate the elbow (skin, muscles, joint
  capsule, ligaments and bony parts)
  while the patient bends, stretches,
  pronates and supinates the arm.

2 Pay special attention to crepitation of
  the humero-ulnar joint.

3 Under pro- and supination, evaluate the
  rotation of the head of the radius (see
  Figure).

4 Lastly, note how the elbow movements
  are performed (smoothly or jerkily).

14.5 Passive movements of the elbow

Purpose

To obtain an impression of the range of movements of the elbow.

Procedure

1 Take hold of the patient's hand with your right hand.

2 Support the patient's upper arm with your left hand (Figure 1).

3 Start carefully to flex the elbow (Figure 2).

4 Evaluate whether and to what extent this is possible.

5 Evaluate the way in which this movement occurs.

6 Perform maximal extension (Figure 3).

7 With the elbow bent, perform pronation and supination (Figure 4).

8 While performing all of these movements, note the degree to which they are possible and how they occur.

9 Pay special attention to any excess mobility, resistance, the cogwheel phenomenon, pain and crepitation.

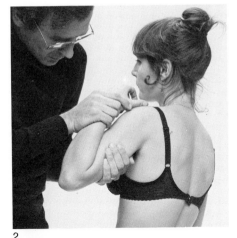

2

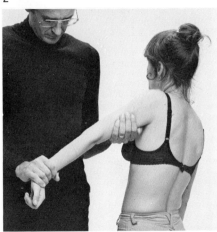

3

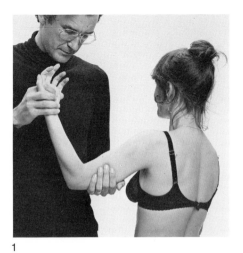

1

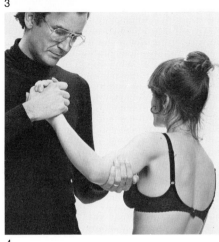

4

D 15 Examination of the wrist, hand and fingers

Purpose
To obtain an impression of the
functioning of the wrist, hand and
fingers.

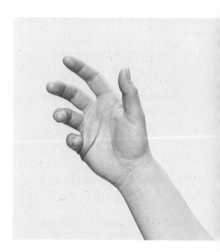

Procedure
1 Ask the patient to expose the arm and
remove all jewelry, etc.

2 Start by inspecting the hands at rest.

3 Inspect active and passive movements
of the hand.

4 Next, palpate the hand at rest and in
movement.

5 Evaluate the functioning of the wrist
and fingers.

6 Compare the right and left hand at each
step.

7 Perform a neurological examination and
assess the peripheral circulation.

15.1 Inspection of the hand at rest

Purpose
To obtain an impression of the shape of
the wrist, hand and fingers.

Procedure

1 The patient should be seated.

2 The patient's forearm is exposed; rings,
 bracelets and the like having been
 removed.

3 Inspect the front and back of the hand
 (Figures 1 and 2).

4 Start with a general inspection, paying
 special attention to:
 - malformations,
 - loss of fingers,
 - defects and anomalies of the position
 in which the hand and fingers are held.

5 Then check the shape of the hand and
 the fingers when the hand is held
 passively, with special attention to:
 - any radial or ulnar deviation,
 - the presence of a "dropped" hand,
 - the presence of a "claw" hand.

6 Next, inspect the skin, noting:
 - color,
 - moistness or dampness of the palm,
 - rigidity,
 - dullness or shininess,
 - edema,
 - scars,
 - contractures,
 - superficial wounds, and
 - any swellings.

7 Inspect the space between the abducted
 thumb and fingers (the anatomical
 'snuff box') (Figure 3).

8 Inspect hair growth and nails.

9 Inspect the contours of the hand.

10 Check for atrophy in the muscles of the
 thumb, little finger or of any of the
 interosseal muscles.

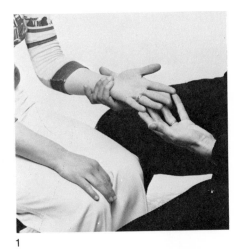

1

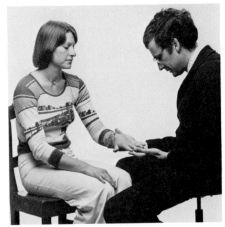

2

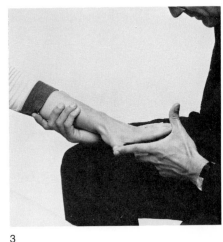

3

227

11 Inspect the contours of the joints, look for:
    - edema,
    - ganglia,
    - cysts,
    - swellings, and
    - inflammation.

12 Inspect the fingers carefully, with special attention to:
    - any contractures,
    - lateral displacement, and
    - swellings.

13 Give extra attention to the tips of the fingers and the nails ('drumstick' fingers, 'spoon'-shaped nails).

Purpose
To form an impression of the shape of
the wrist, the hand and the fingers by
palpation.

Procedure
1 Start with a general inspection.

2 The hand must be as relaxed as
   possible during palpation.

3 Attempt to obtain information about the
   condition of the skin, the musculature
   and the tendon sheaths while palpating.

4 Palpate the skin over the various joints
   (e.g. temperature, mobility, and
   swellings; Figure 1).

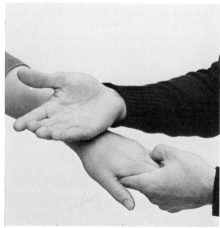

1

5 Palpate the muscles around the various
   joints (tone, sensitivity to pain, and any
   firm or hard swellings).

6 Then give special attention to the wrist
   and any swelling in this region (e.g.
   carpal ganglion).

7 Palpate the wrist ligaments.

8 Palpate the tendon sheaths on the back
   of the hand (Figure 2).

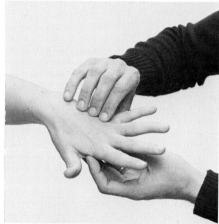

9 In the palm, palpate the tendon sheaths
   and the palmar aponeurosis.

2

10 Next, palpate the bones of the wrist,
   hand and fingers (Figure 3), with special
   attention to:
   - thickening,
   - pain,
   - or deviant position.

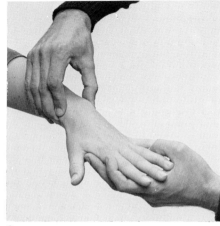

3

11 Palpate the anatomical 'snuff box' (Figure 4).

12 Lastly, palpate the finger joints, noting swelling, inflammation, edema, and the condition of the joint capsule.

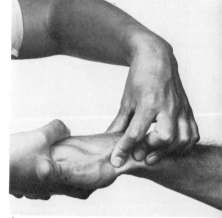

4

Purpose

To form an impression of the functioning of the wrist, hand and fingers, by inspection.

Procedure

1 Ask the patient to perform a number of active movements (Figures 1–11):
   - to stretch and bend the wrist,
   - to turn the wrist to each side,
   - to spread and close the fingers,
   - to bend the stretched fingers at the metacarpophalangeal joint,
   - to bend these fingers further and also at the interphalangeal joint until the tips reach the palm,
   - to bend the fingers one by one with the others extended,
   - to touch the tip of the thumb with the tip of each of the other fingers successively,
   - with the thumb stretched, to bend and stretch the thumb.

2 Note whether, and if so to what extent, these movements can be performed.

3 Compare right and left at each step.

4 Lastly, assess the power of all movements by asking the patient to perform them while you apply resistance.

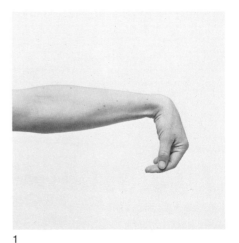

1

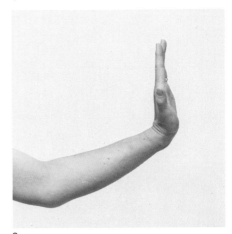

2

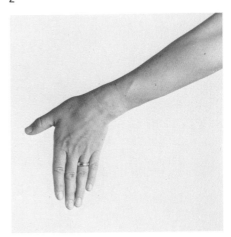

3

231

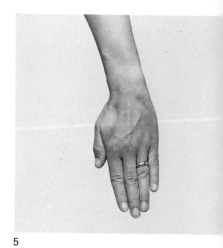

5

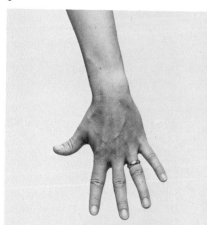

6

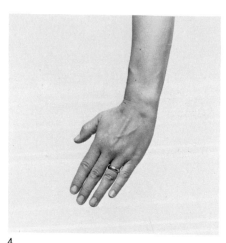

4

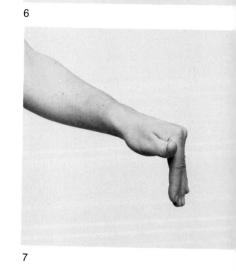

7

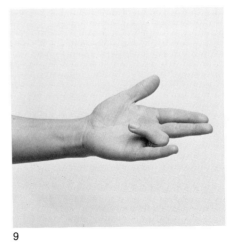

9

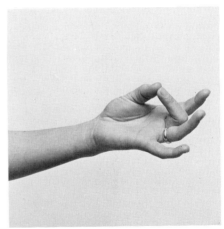

10

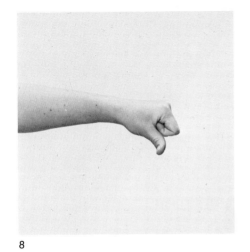

8

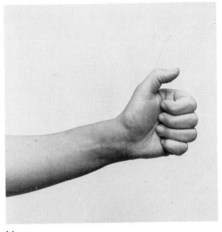

11

D 15.4 Palpation of the moving hand

Purpose
To perform an impression of the functioning of the wrist, hand and fingers by means of palpation.

Procedure

1. Ask the patient to perform all possible movements with the wrist, hand and fingers (see D 15.3).

2. Start by palpating the movements in the wrist (flexion, extension, adduction and abduction).

3. Note whether, and to what extent, these movements are performed.

4. Palpate the dorsal and ventral sides in particular (e.g. ganglion, carpal tunnel syndrome).

5. Then palpate the palm of the hand.

6. Evaluate any pain on compression of the metacarpals (Figure 1).

7. Assess the sensitivity of the bones of the fingers to pressure (Figure 2).

8. Lastly, palpate the metacarpo-phalangeal and interphalangeal joints under maximal extension and maximal flexion (Figures 3 and 4).

9. Check for swelling of these joints.

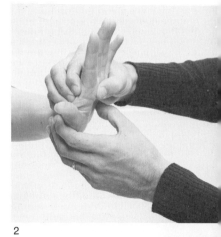

2

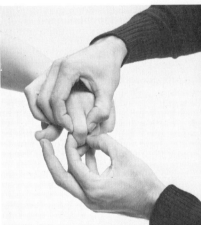

3

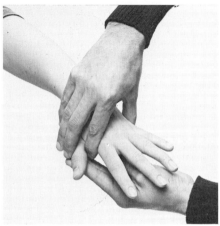

1

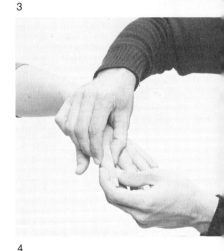

4

Purpose
To obtain an impression of the mobility of the hand.

Procedure

1 Examine the wrist joint first.

2 Support the patient's forearm with one of your hands and surround the patient's hand with your other hand.

3 Bend the hand backwards (maximal extension of the wrist; Figure 1).

4 Then perform maximal flexion (Figure 2).

5 Evaluate adduction and abduction (Figures 3 and 4).

6 Continue your examination by flexing and extending each of the metacarpophalangeal joints.

7 Then do the same for the proximal interphalangeal joints and lastly for the distal interphalangeal joints (Figures 5 and 6).

8 Examine the passive mobility of the wrist.

9 Note whether, and if so to what extent, these movements can be performed.

10 Note how these movements occur (smoothly, stiffly, painfully, etc.).

11 Pay special attention to:
   - excess or restricted mobility,
   - resistance,
   - crepitation,
   - pain.

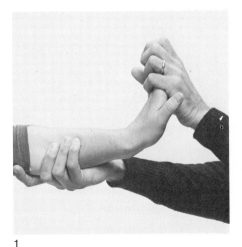

1

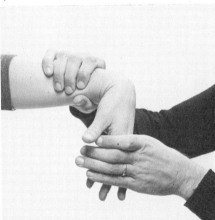

2

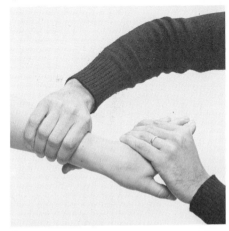

3

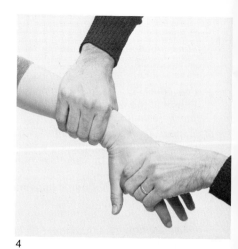

4

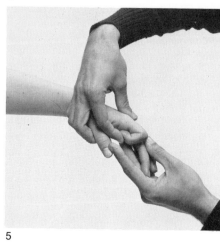

5

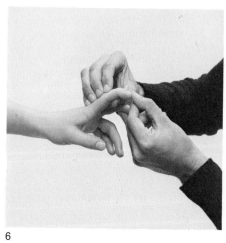

6

236

Purpose
To obtain an impression of the shape and functioning of the leg.

Procedure
1 Ask the patient to undress from the waist down, including the feet.

2 Begin the inspection; perform it systematically.

3 Inspect the front, back and sides of the leg.

4 Compare the right and left leg.

5 Inspect with the patient lying down, standing and moving (walking).

6 Start by inspecting the hips.

7 Supplement your inspection with palpation of the hips and an evaluation of their function.

8 Examine the knee in the same way.

9 Inspect and palpate the ankle.

10 Next, evaluate ankle and foot function.

11 If appropriate, evaluate the peripheral arterial circulation (D 16.1).

12 If appropriate, do the same for the venous circulation (D 16.2).

13 If appropriate, measure the circumference of the upper and/or lower leg.

14 Lastly, perform a neurological examination of the leg (C 5).

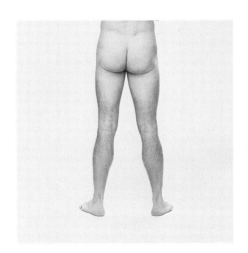

D 16.1 Peripheral circulation in the leg

Purpose
To form an impression of the quality of the peripheral arterial vascular system or circulation (Figure 1).

Procedure

1 The legs should be bare.

2 Compare the right and left legs throughout.

3 Start by inspecting the skin.

4 Note any colour changes in the resting leg.

5 Note any colour changes at elevation of the leg:
   - the patient is supine,
   - ask the patient to raise the stretched legs (90° at the hip),
   - note colour changes in this position,
   - note colour changes after the patient has 'cycled' for 2 minutes,
   - note colour changes after the patient has resumed the supine position, and estimate the rate at which the colour returns (left and right),
   - ask the patient to sit up and dangle the legs; note any bluish-red discolorations.

6 Also note:
   - colour changes when the hands and feet cool,
   - trophic disorders with evidence of ulceration, infection, or
   - visible arterial pulsations,
   - hyperhydrosis.

7 Palpate and assess successively:
   - temperature of both legs (differences),
   - the femoral, popliteal and posterior tibial arteries and the dorsal digital artery of the foot (Figures 2–5),
   - during this palpation, note the condition of the vessel wall (normally not palpable, margins imprecise, vessel easily compressed and elastic),
   - evaluate the pulse.

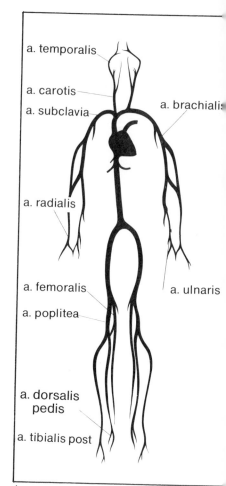

a. temporalis
a. carotis
a. subclavia
a. brachialis
a. radialis
a. femoralis
a. poplitea
a. dorsalis pedis
a. tibialis post
a. ulnaris

1

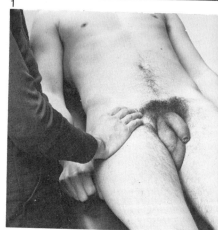

2

8 Auscultate the femoral artery. Note:
- the number of sounds per beat,
- vascular murmurs,
- regularity of the rhythm,
- equality of the pulsations.

9 If appropriate, determine the claudication distance.

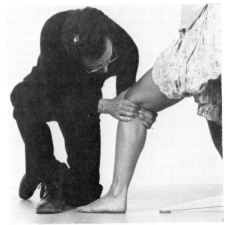

3

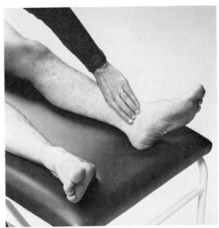

4

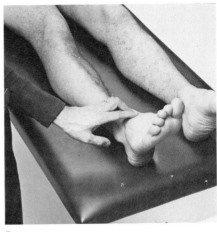

5

D 16.2 Examination of the veins

Purpose
To obtain an impression of the shape
and functioning of the veins in the leg
and the quality of the venous circulation.

Procedure
• The examination of the veins is always
part of another examination.

1 The legs should be bare.

2 Have good illumination.

3 Compare the right and left sides at each
step.

4 During inspection, look for:
 - varices in the course of the saphenous
   veins,
 - thrombophlebitis
 - edema,
 - varicose ulcers or the scars of such
   ulcers,
 - shiny skin,
 - discoloration (i.e. cyanosis),
 - scaling,
 - pigmentations.

5 Next, palpate the varices. Note any
swellings, pain and warmth due to
inflammation.

6 Palpate edema, if any; find out whether
pitting edema is present.

7 Palpate the calf muscles. Check for
pressure pain in the calf.
 • Pressure pain can be appreciably more
 severe under dorsiflexion of the foot.

8 Next, perform auscultation (of minor
importance for the venous circulation).

9 Lastly, perform specific function tests
when superficial varices are present.

Test A

10 - the patient stands erect,
   - place a tourniquet above the varicosity such that the peripheral arteries are still just palpable,
   - ask the patient to walk around for a while; complete emptying of the varicosity indicates a patent deep venous system and competence of the valves in the perforating veins.

Test B

11 - the patient lies down and raises the legs to allow the varicosities to empty;
   - compress the saphenous vein by applying a tourniquet at the thigh or under the knee;
   - have the patient stand up;
   - note how the saphenous vein fills, i.e. slowly (after about 30 seconds, indicating competence of the valves of the perforating veins) or rapidly (incompetence of the valves of the perforating veins),
   - release the tourniquet: if the varicosity fills distalward, the valves of the saphenous vein are not competent.

D 16.3 Measurement of the circumference of the leg

Purpose

To obtain an impression of any atrophy or hypertrophy by measurement of the circumference of the upper or lower leg.

Procedure

1 The legs and the area just above them should be exposed.

2 Ask the patient to sit down with legs spread apart.

3 Determine the midpoint between the anterior superior spine and the upper edge of the patella (Figure 1).

4 Mark this point.

5 On the lower leg, find the widest part of the calf and mark that (Figure 2).

6 Measure with the tapemeasure perpendicular to the longitudinal axis of the leg and passing over the marked points (Figure 3).

7 Record the circumference to an accuracy of 0.1 cm.

8 Compare the right and left leg.

9 The circumference of the upper leg is often measured in another way as well: by starting with the determination of the midline of the knee joint,

10 and then marking off points 20 cm higher and 15 cm lower,

11 measure the circumference over these marked points and perpendicular to the long axis of the leg.

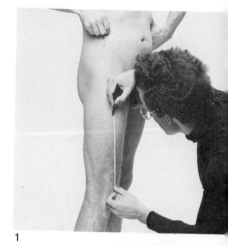

1

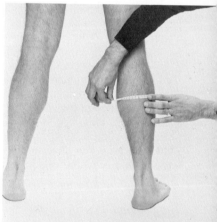

2

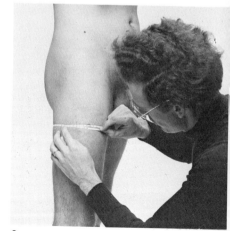

3

16.4 Evaluation of the gait

Purpose
To obtain an impression, by inspection, of the way in which walking movements are performed.

Procedure

1 Ask the patient to walk (see Figure).

2 Inspect the gait from the front, the sides, and the back.

3 Attempt to analyse the various phases of locomotion.

4 During these phases inspect for any changes in the movements of the hip joints, the knees, and the ankles.
- First phase:
  hip: slight anteflexion → retroflexion,
  knee: slightly bent → bent further → extended,
  ankle: limited dorsal flexion → plantar flexion.

- Second phase:
  hip: retroflexion → anteflexion,
  knee: extended → slightly bent,
  ankle: plantar flexion → dorsal flexion → pelvis tipped forward.
- Attempt to obtain an impression of the ease with which a normal gait is achieved.

5 Pay attention to the movements of the other parts of the body during walking, particularly those of the hips, the vertebral column and the head.

6 Note how the patient moves the arms while walking.

7 Important information can be obtained by inspecting the soles of the patient's shoes (degree and pattern of wear).

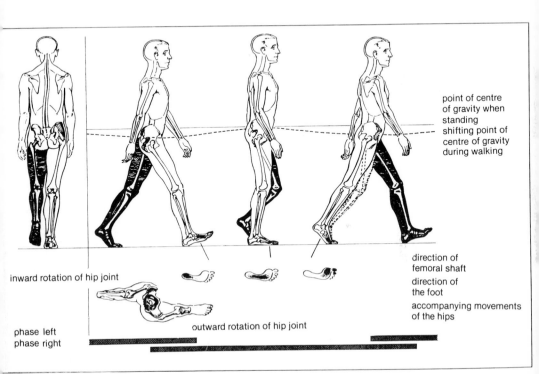

point of centre of gravity when standing
shifting point of centre of gravity during walking

direction of femoral shaft
direction of the foot
accompanying movements of the hips

inward rotation of hip joint

outward rotation of hip joint

phase left
phase right

(From Lohman, A. H. M. (1977). *Vorm en beweging* (Form and movement). 4th ed., (Utrecht)

D 17   Examination of the hip

Purpose
To obtain an impression of the shape and functioning of the hip.

Procedure
- Examination of the hips is almost always combined with an examination of the back.
- The back and hip examinations are usually part of the examination for muscular function.
- Neurological examination of the hip is restricted to the evaluation of muscle power.

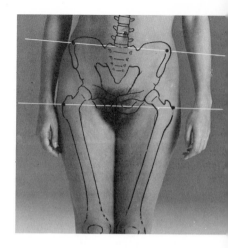

1 The patient should undress.

2 Start with inspection of the hips while the patient stands. (Check for tilting of the pelvis; see Figure)

3 Attempt to obtain additional information about the hips by palpation.

4 Ask the patient to perform a number of movements (while standing and lying down).

5 Evaluate the passive movements of the hip joint.

6 Lastly, perform a special function test (D 11.6).

7 Compare the right and left side at each step.

8 Perform a neurological examination and examine the arterial circulation.

Purpose
To form an impression of the shape and
stance of the hips and pelvis.

Procedure
1 The patient should be standing relaxed,
with the feet together and the legs
straight or lying on a flat firm surface.

2 Inspect all four sides.

3 Inspect the skin over the joint
(discoloration, swelling, scars,
inflammation).

4 Pay special attention to the skin folds
(Figures 1 and 2). Are the buttock folds
symmetrical? Are there extra folds? Is
the fold of the groin depressed? Is the
cleft between the buttocks straight?

5 Inspect the contours of the joint.
 • Orientation points are provided by the
greater trochanters, the iliac crests and
the anterior and posterior iliac spines.

6 Check for joint swelling.

7 Note the position or posture of the
vertebral column:
 - in the supine patient,
 - in the standing patient.

8 Note the position of the hips.
 • Orientation points: the anterior superior
iliac spines, the greater trochanters and
the line between the greater trochanters.

9 Note the position of the legs.
 • Orientation points are provided by the
greater trochanters, the patellae and the
position of the feet as well as the
outline of the space between the legs.

10 Note the appearance of the upper leg
(atrophy or hypertrophy).

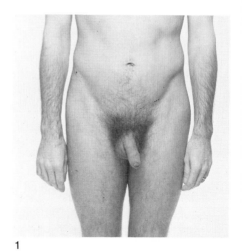

1

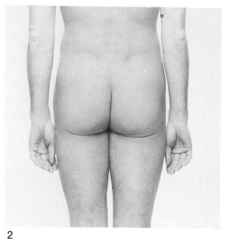

2

D 17.2 Palpation of the hip at rest

Purpose
To collect supplementary information about the shape of the hip.

Procedure
1 Palpate the skin over the joint (temperature, mobility, swelling; (Figure 1).

2 Palpate the muscles around the joint (tone, atrophy, pain, swellings).

3 Palpate the joint capsule (Figures 2 and 3) by:
- palpating from the ventral direction,
- palpating from the lateral direction (behind the great trochanter).

4 Palpate the bony parts of the joint.

5 Palpate the nerves around the joint to find the neurological 'pressure points' of the sciatic, femoral and obturator nerves (Figures 3 and 4).

6 Palpate the lymph glands in the groin as well.

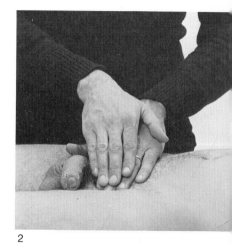

2

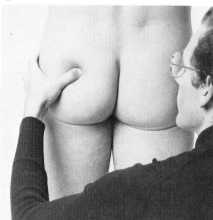

3

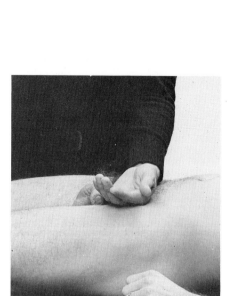

1

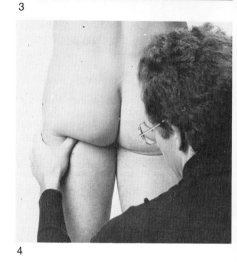

4

D 17.3 Inspection of the active movements of the hip

Purpose
To obtain an impression of the range of active movements of the hip.

Procedure
1 The patient should be lying supine.

2 Ask the patient to flex the hips (with extended leg and with flexed knee, Figures 1 and 2).

3 Evaluate abduction and adduction as well.

4 Evaluate inward and outward rotation (Figures 3 and 4).

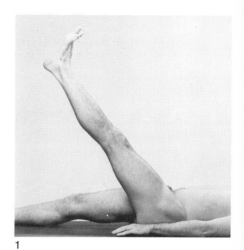

1

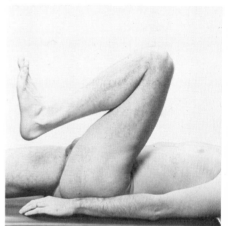

2

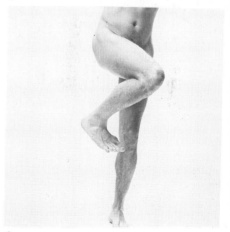

3

5 Ask the patient to turn over.

6 In the prone position, evaluate the range of extension and flexion (Figure 5).

7 Ask the patient to stand up.

8 For each leg, ask the patient to raise the knee as high as possible and to swing it to the left and right as far as possible (Figure 4).

9 Note whether he can do so and to what degree.

10 Also note how the movement is performed (smoothly, stiffly, painfully or cautiously).

11 Assess the strength of all movements by asking the patient to perform them against the resistance of your hands.

12 Ask the patient to walk back and forth.

13 Note whether the stepping distance is the same for both legs.

14 Estimate whether the same load is put on both legs.

15 Note whether the associated movements of the vertebral column are smooth.

16 Lastly, ask the patient to walk on tiptoe and then on the heels.

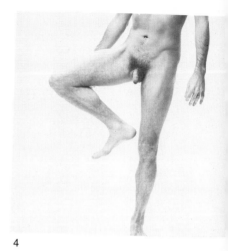

4

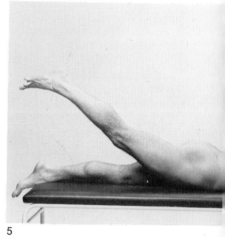

5

Purpose
To obtain an impression of the course
of the hip movements.

Procedure
1 The patient is asked to lie flat on the
   examining table.

2 Ask him to perform the following
   movements successively:
   - adduction,
   - abduction,
   - inward rotation (with flexed knee),
   - outward rotation (with flexed knee),
   - flexion,
   - extension (with flexed and extended
     knee).

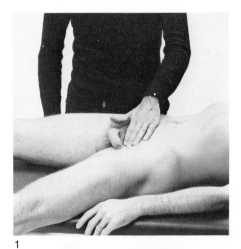

1

3 While each movement is being made,
   palpate the hip joint in the fold of the
   groin (Figures 1 and 2).

4 Evaluate the smoothness of the
   movements and watch for crepitation
   and pressure pain.

5 Palpate the musculature around the
   joint as well.

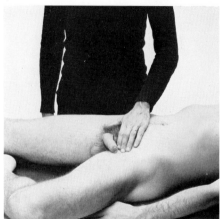

2

249

D 17.5 Passive movements of the hip

Purpose

To obtain an impression of the range of movements of the hip joint.

Procedure

1 The patient is placed on the back on a firm surface.

2 Grasp with one hand the foot on the side of the hip to be examined.

3 Support the upper leg with your other hand.

4 Start to bend the hip carefully (Figures 1 and 2).

5 This is often easiest to do if the knee if maximally flexed.

6 Next, perform outward and inward rotation with the knee flexed 90° and the hip flexed 90° (Figures 3 and 4).

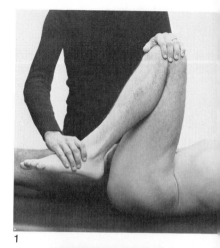
1

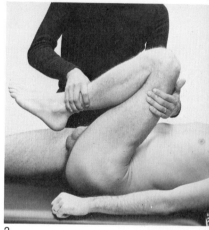
2

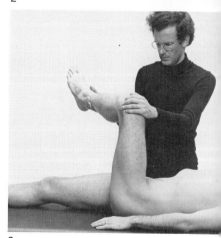
3

7 Evaluate the abduction and adduction range of the hip (with the leg stretched).

8 With the patient lying prone, passive extension and flexion can be evaluated in the same way (Figure 5).

9 In each case judge the extent to which the movement is possible.

10 Judge how these movements occur.

11 Note whether these movements cause pain and/or crepitation.

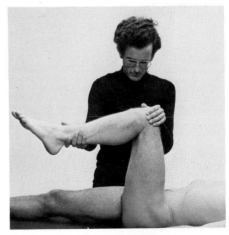

4

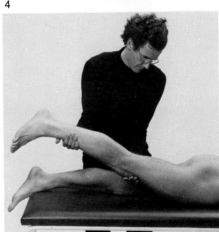

5

D 17.6 Some specific hip function tests

Purpose

To obtain information about the functioning of the hips by performing specific tests.

Procedure

A

1 Ask the patient to stand up.

2 Ask the patient to lift one leg with bent knee ('stork' position: Figure 1).

3 Note whether this causes the hip to drop on that side (Figure 2).
 • This test detects the gluteal muscles' competence.

B

1 The patient should lie supine on the examining table.

2 Check whether lumbar lordosis is present.

3 Bend the hip and the knee such that the lordosis disappears.

4 Pay special attention to the upper part of the other leg (Figure 3).
 • If it moves upward at the same time in the hip area, there must be a flexion contracture on that side.

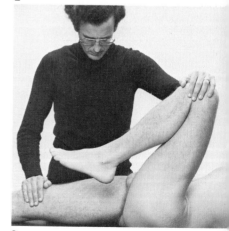

1

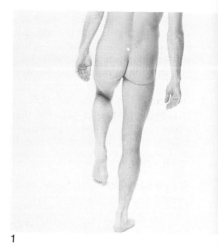

2

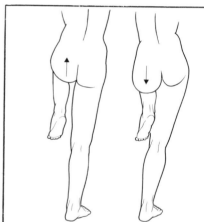

3

C

1 Measure the anatomical length (distance between the great trochanter and the lateral malleolus) (Figure 4).

2 Determine the clinical length (distance between the anterior superior iliac spine − measured over the inner edge of the patella − and the middle malleolus) (Figure 5).

3 Before you start to measure, be sure the patient's pelvis is lying straight.

D

● Apply this test for the detection of a congenitally dislocated hip in a newborn.

1 Place the baby on its back.

2 Grasp the lower legs just under the knee (Figure 6).

3 Then attempt to abduct and outwardly rotate each of the flexed hips (Figure 7).

4 If you feel or hear a click, the test result is positive and congenital dislocation of a hip is probable.

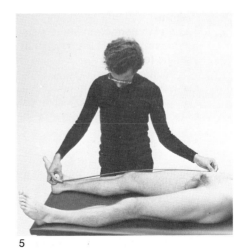

5

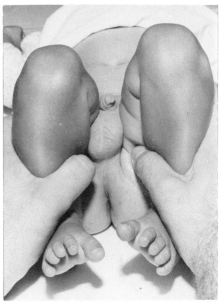

6

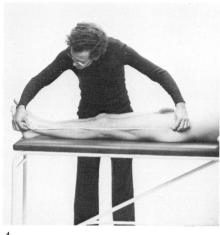

4

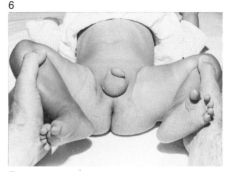

7

Figures 6 and 7 from Kingma, M. J. (1979). (Ed.). *Netherlands Handbook on Orthopaedics.* 3rd ed. (Utrecht)

D 18   Examination of the knee

Purpose
To obtain an impression of the shape
and functioning of the knee joint.

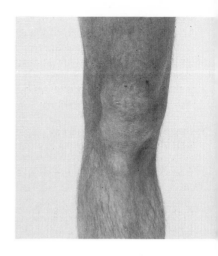

Procedure
- The knee examination usually forms
  part of the examination for effective
  movement or mobility (mainly the feet,
  hips and back).

1 Ask the patient to expose the legs.

2 Compare the right and left leg
   throughout.

3 Remember that the knee has a back and
   sides as well.

4 Examine the patient both standing and
   lying down.

5 Examine the patient at rest and moving.

6 Start with a close inspection.

7 Palpation of the knee supplies valuable
   supplementary information.

8 Assess the mobility range of the knee
   both actively and passively.

9 Perform a number of function tests:
   - assess the mobility of the menisci,
   - assess any excessive mobility of the
     anterior cruciate ligament,
   - assess lateral mobility of the lateral
     ligaments.

10 If appropriate, measure the
    circumference of the upper leg to obtain
    an indication of possible atrophy of the
    quadriceps.

11 Perform a neurological examination and
    examine the peripheral circulation.

8.1 Inspection of the knee at rest

Purpose
To obtain an impression of the shape and position of the knee at rest.

Procedure
1 Ask the patient to lie down on his back with the legs flat and relaxed.

2 Inspect the knee from the front and sides (see Figure).

3 Compare the right and left knee at each step.

4 Inspect the skin around the joint (discoloration, swelling, scars).

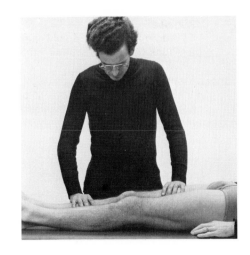

5 Note the contours of the knee and any deviation in position held.
   ● Orientation points are provided by the medial and lateral epicondyles of the femur, the patella, the tibial tuberosity, the medial condyle of the tibia and the head of the fibula.

6 Look for signs of fluid in the knee joint (indistinct contours, disappearance of the normal recesses above). If necessary, measure the circumference of the knee.

7 Note any swelling of the suprapatellar, prepatellar, and/or infrapatellar bursae.

8 Note the appearance of the upper and lower legs (atrophy or hypertrophy). Measure the circumference of the upper and lower legs.

9 With the patient still supine, supplement your examination with palpation of the knee.

10 Ask the patient to stand relaxed with the feet slightly apart.

11 Inspect all four sides of the knee.

12 Here too, pay special attention to the skin, contours and any swellings.

13 Give extra attention to the position the knee is held in (valgus, varus, or hyperextension).
   ● Orientation points: middle of kneecap, middle of ankle joint, head of the third metatarsal) and the knee folds.

D 18.2 Palpation of the knee at rest

Purpose

To obtain information, by palpation, about the shape and any abnormalities of the shape of the knee.

Procedure

● Palpation should be combined with inspection throughout.

1 Ask the patient to lie down and relax.

2 Palpate with the knee dangling as well.

3 Start by palpating the skin over the joint: temperature (judged with the back of the hand), mobility, swellings (Figure 1).

4 Palpate the muscles around the joint (tone, atrophy, pain, swellings; Figure 2).

5 Palpate the joint capsule between the medial epicondyle of the femur, the medial condyle of the tibia, and the medial ligament (Figure 3).

6 Palpate the bony parts of the knee:
- the patella,
- the femoral condyles, first medially and then laterally,
- the tibial condyles, first medially and then laterally,
- the tuberosity of the tibia,
- the head of the fibula.

7 Palpate the joint groove as well.

8 The back of the knee is palpated most easily when the patient is either standing or lying down with the knee slightly flexed.

9 Palpate the arteries:
- the popliteal artery in relation to
- the femoral artery,
- the posterior tibial artery, and
- the dorsal artery of the foot.

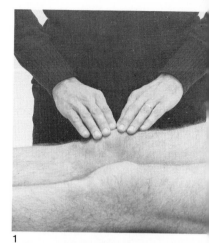

1

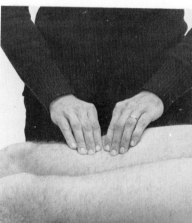

2

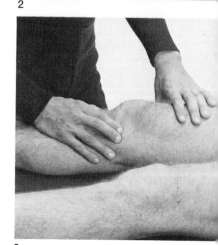

3

10 Palpation at rest is concluded with
   examination of the patella for mobility
   and the presence of fluid:
   - press the superior aspect of the
     recess above the patella to empty it
     by putting one hand around the upper
     leg just above the patella and pressing
     any fluid present downwards to bring
     it under the patella (Figures 4 and 5),
   - with the index finger of the other hand,
     press the patella inwards.
   ● If the patella moves backwards and
     forwards against resistance then fluid is
     present in the knee joint.

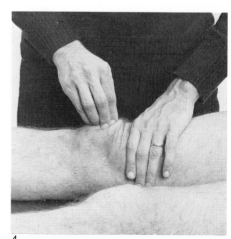

4

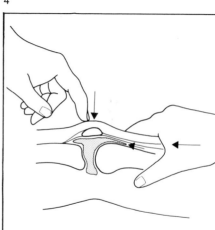

5

D 18.3 Inspection of the active movements of the knee

Purpose
To obtain an impression of the range of active movements of the knee.

Procedure
1 Ask the patient to lie down and bend the knees as much as possible (Figure 1).

2 Judge whether and to what degree this is possible and how the movement is performed (smoothly, with pain, etc.).

3 With the knee bent as far as the patient can, assess the outline of the space between the calf and the upper leg on both sides (Figure 2).

4 Check whether the heels are aligned to the hips (Figure 3).

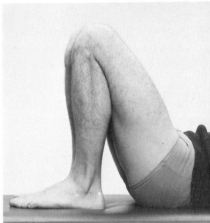

1

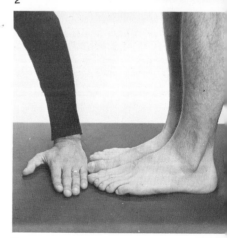

2

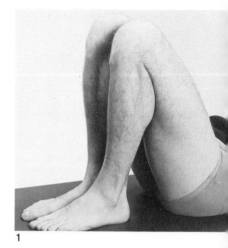

3

5 Note whether the knees are at the same height (Figure 4).

6 Ask the patient to stretch the legs, if possible more than 180°.

7 Note whether this is possible, and if so to what degree and how this movement is performed.

8 Then ask the patient to stand up.

9 Ask the patient to squat on his heels (Figure 5).

10 Make a similar evaluation.

11 Ask the patient to walk.

12 Note in particular whether the knee movements are smooth.

13 Lastly, assess the strength of all of these movements by having the patient perform them against resistance.

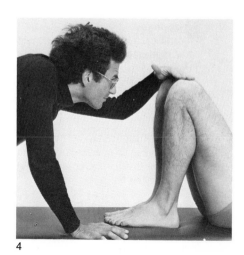
4

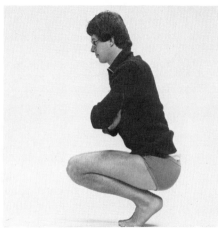
5

D 18.4 Palpation of the moving knee

Purpose

To obtain an impression of the course of the knee movements.

Procedure

● Palpation during movement is always supplementary to inspection.

1 Ask the patient to lie down.

2 Ask the patient to repeatedly bend and stretch the knee.

3 Place the palm of your hand on the patella (Figure 1).

4 Judge how the movement is performed.

5 Note whether this flexion—extension movement proceeds smoothly.

6 Note coarse or fine crepitation.

7 During the same movements, palpate the various bursae and joint fissures (Figure 2).

8 Watch for swellings and pressure pain sensitivity.

9 Ask the patient to flex the foot 90° and then to outward and inward rotate it (Figure 3).

10 Lastly, palpate the joint fissure with respect to swelling or sensitivity for pressure pain.

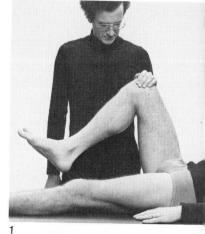

1

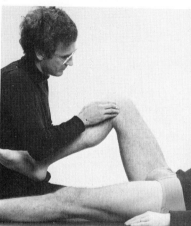

2

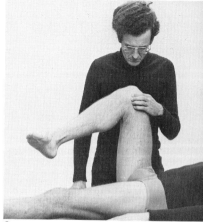

3

D 18.5 Passive movements of the knee

Purpose
To obtain an impression of the range of passive movements of the knee.

Procedure
1 Ask the patient to lie down in the supine position.

2 Grasp the ankle firmly.

3 Bring the ankle carefully toward the patient's buttock (flexion of the knee) (Figure 1).

4 Judge whether and, if so, to what extent this is possible (mobility range) and how it occurs (smoothly, painfully etc.).

5 With the same grip, bring the knee into the extended position (Figure 2).

6 During both flexion and extension, attempt to differentiate between functional restrictions due to pain or to any anatomical abnormalities.

7 Next, assess the adduction and abduction ranges of the knee (examination of the collateral ligaments, D 18.6).

8 Lastly, assess the range of inward and outward rotation (lower leg relative to upper leg) with the knee flexed (Figure 3).

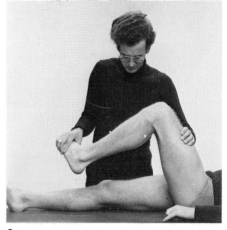

1

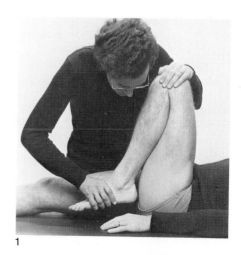

2

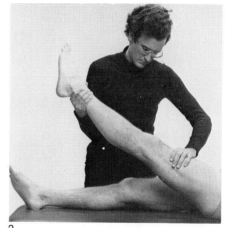

3

D 18.6 Some specific knee function tests

Purpose

To obtain information about the condition of the menisci, the cruciate ligaments and the collateral ligaments.

Procedure

A Examination of the menisci

1 Place your finger tips on the medial side of the joint fissure with the knee bent as much as possible (Figure 1).

2 Outwardly rotate the lower leg for the examination of the medial meniscus (Figure 1).

3 Then stretch the knee while palpating the medial fissure with your finger tips (Figure 2).

4 Then bend the knee back to the 90° flexion position.

5 While doing this, have your finger tips on the lateral fissure.

6 Inwardly rotate the lower leg and ask the patient to stretch the leg slowly.

7 If you feel or hear a click during extension or the patient shows that this is painful, the test result is positive.

B Examination of the cruciate ligaments

1 The patient is supine.

2 The leg to be examined is flexed to 90°.

3 Fix the foot of that leg securely, e.g. by sitting on it.

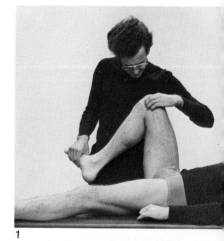

1

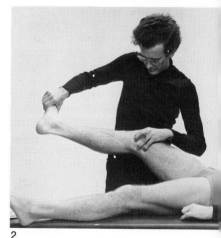

2

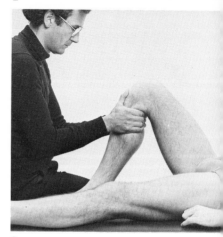

3

4 With both hands, take hold of the lower leg firmly just below the knee and palpate the patella with your thumbs.

5 Attempt to draw the lower leg forward (thus testing the anterior cruciate) and then backward (thus testing the posterior cruciate; Figure 3).

6 When anomalies are found, defects in the cruciate ligaments are considered to be present.

C Examination of the collateral ligaments (for lateral mobility)

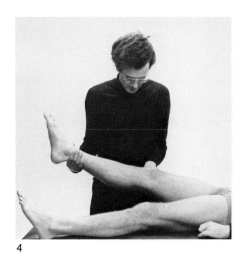

4

1 The patient lies supine with the legs completely stretched.

2 Grasp one ankle medially with one hand and put your other hand around the upper leg laterally just above the knee.

3 Next, apply opposing pressure briefly with your hands (thus testing the medial ligaments; Figure 4).

4 With the pressures exerted in the opposite direction, the lateral ligaments are tested.

D 19   Examination of the ankle, foot and toes

Purpose
To obtain an impression of the shape and functioning of the ankles, feet and toes.

Procedure
1 Ask the patient to remove any clothing covering the legs and feet.

2 Start by inspecting the structures at rest with the patient standing, sitting and lying down.

3 Next, inspect the feet while the patient performs active movements, e.g. while walking and/or sitting.

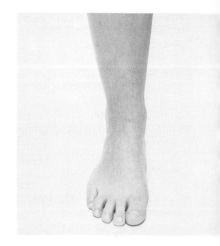

4 Continue the examination with palpation at rest and during movement.

5 With the help of your findings, determine the state of the function of the individual joints.

6 Examine the circulation.

7 Perform a neurological examination.

8 Compare right and left.

19.1 Inspection of the ankle, foot and toes at rest

Purpose
To obtain an impression of the ankles, feet and toes at rest.

Procedure

1 The patient stands relaxed on both feet.

2 Ask the patient to place the feet 15–20 centimeters apart (Figure 1).

3 Inspect the feet from the front, from the sides and from the back.

4 Note any deviation in the shape or position of the foot.

5 Pay special attention to the arches, the width of the foot and the toes (Figure 2).

6 Inspect the shape of the ankle and the foot.

7 Note whether the rear aspect of the foot (calcaneum) is straight under the lower leg (Figure 3).
   • Deviations are often due to, for instance, deformities of the knee joint.

8 Check for a deformity in the position of the forefoot.

9 Note the shape of the toes (hallux valgus; Figure 4).

10 Continue your inspection with close scrutiny of the toe nails and the skin of the foot.

11 Look in particular for swellings (abnormal callus formation, or any bony projections) and for varicosities.

12 Pay special attention to the color of the skin and toe nails.

13 Do not forget the areas between the toes (for skin diseases etc.).

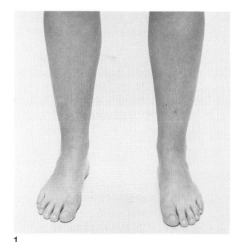

1

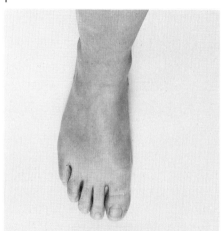

2

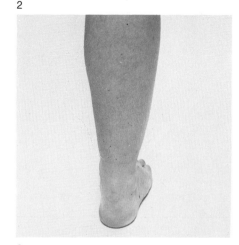

3

265

14 Ask the patient to sit on the edge of the examining table with the legs dangling.

15 Pay special attention to the position of the foot relative to the lower leg.

16 Ask the patient to lie down on the examining table.

17 Inspect the weight-bearing parts of the feet first (Figure 5).

18 Look in particular for signs of hyperkeratosis and any callus formation.

19 Inspect the vault of the arch.

20 Note any muscle atrophy and swellings.

21 Compare the right and left side throughout.

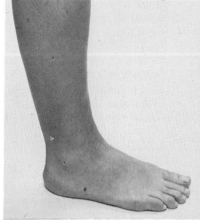

4

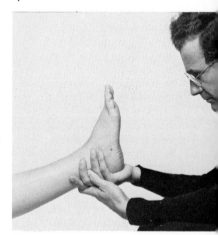

5

D 19.2 Palpation of the ankle, foot and toes at rest

Purpose
To obtain an impression of the shape (or malformation) of the ankles, feet and toes.

Procedure
1 Palpate any abnormalities found at inspection of the ankle and foot.

2 While palpating any swelling, note in particular:
   - the consistency,
   - size,
   - extension,
   - relationship with the surrounding tissues,
   - temperature (Figure 1).

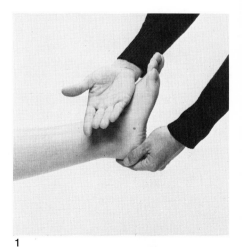

1

3 While palpating the foot joints look for signs of edema, or fluctuation of the left and right extensor tendon movements.

4 Assess the quality of the ankle joint capsules.

5 Pay special attention to the temperature (use the back of your hand) and the peripheral circulation (dorsal artery of the foot and posterior tibial artery; Figure 2).

6 Compare left and right throughout.

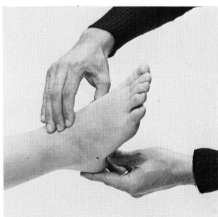

2

D 19.3 Inspection of the active movements of the ankle, foot and toes

Purpose
To form an impression of the range of active movement of the ankles, feet and toes.

Procedure
1 The lower limbs are exposed and allow room for movement.

2 Inspect the gait and the positions the foot is put through (i.e. walking pattern, lameness, limping, rolling or any other defects).

3 Inspect the way in which the foot is placed on the floor and the phases of the gait (Figures 1 and 2).

4 Note whether the patient lifts the feet or shuffles.

5 Note inversion of the feet, or eversion of the feet.
  ●Abnormalities of the feet or gait are often caused by abnormalities in other muscles of the lower limb or in its enervation.

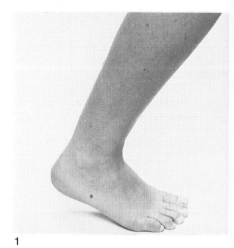

1

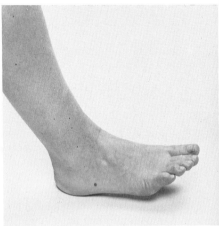

2

6 Ask the patient to walk rapidly.

7 Ask the patient to walk on toes and then on the heels (Figures 3 and 4).

8 After that, ask the patient to walk on the insides and outsides of the feet (Figures 5 and 6).

9 Lastly, evaluate the power of all movements of the ankle and foot by having the sitting patient perform them while you attempt to impede the movement with your hands.

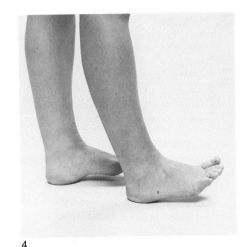

4

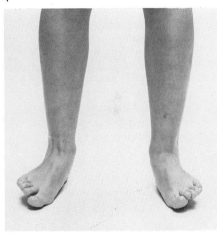

5

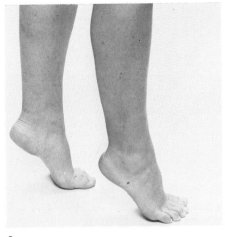

3

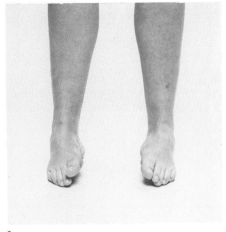

6

D 19.4 Palpation of the moving ankle, foot and toes

Purpose
To form an impression of the course of the foot movements.

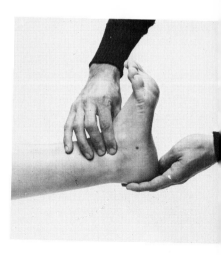

Procedure
1 Ask the patient to lie down and relax.

2 Ask the patient to perform all movements of the ankle, foot and toes.

3 Palpate the foot during all of these movements.

4 Pay special attention to the various joint movements and mobility of the ligaments, the muscles and the tendons (see Figure).

5 Note how these movements are performed.

6 Pay special attention to crepitation and pain (under pressure or during movement).

7 If the foot is flat, check whether this can be corrected.

Purpose
To obtain an impression of the range of passive movements of the foot.

Procedure
1 Start with the passive movements of the ankle joint.

2 For this purpose, hold the patient's leg still with one hand and with the other hand grasp the middle of that foot.

3 Perform the following movements:
- plantar and dorsal flexion (Figures 1 and 2),
- inversion (a combination of plantar flexion, adduction, and supination; Figure 3),
- eversion (a combination of dorsal flexion, abduction, and pronation),
- the movements of the forefoot (minimal plantar and dorsal flexion).

4 Inspect the passive movements of the toes (Figure 4).

5 Note how the movements are performed and whether restriction of movement is present.

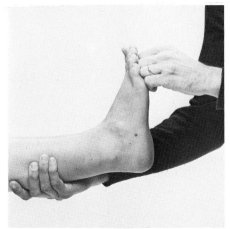

2

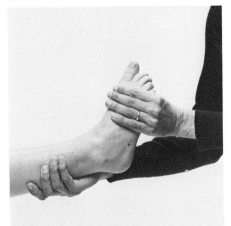

3

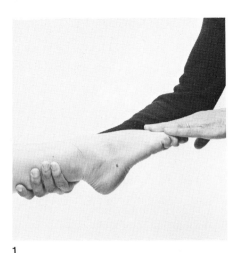

1

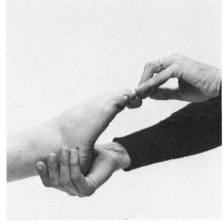

4

Index

278